Budwig Protocol

Cancer Cure is possible

Dedication

I dedicate this book to your Mom, how much you suffered from cancer and I could not save you.

I dedicate this book to you my darling Usha for your kindness, devotion, and making wonderful oil-protein muesli whenever I needed energy. You witnesses every moment of making this book.

I dedicate this book to you my sweet Aishvarya for encouragement and endless support you gave me at every step of making this book.

I also dedicate this book to my close friends and relatives Dr. B.L.Gochar, my sister Urmila, Mr. Pradeep Ladiwal, Mr. Vijay Seth, Mr. Jayanti Jain and Mr. Anil Paul for inspiring me to write this book.

I am thankful to Mr. Allan Cortez and Dr. Arun Nema who helped me for making corrections, typos and suggestions.

Dr. Om Verma

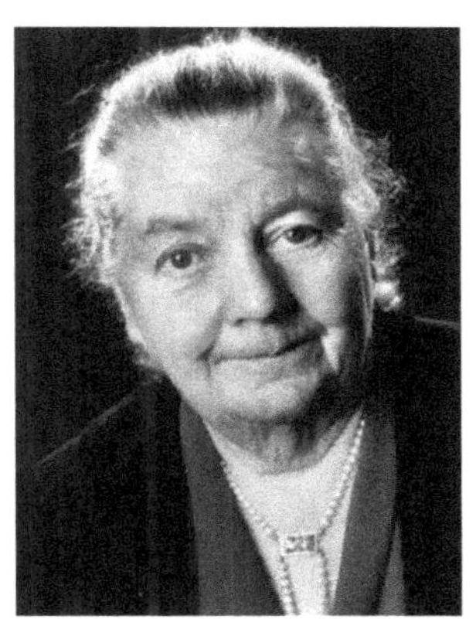

Dr. Johanna Budwig
(30 Sept, 1908 - 19 May, 2003)
Seven Time Nobel Prize Nominee
Known as Omega-3 Lady
90% Documented Success

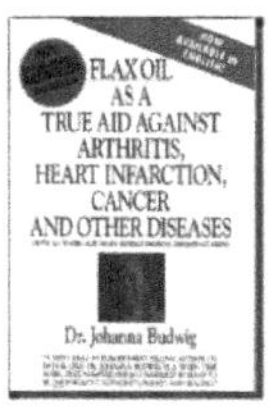

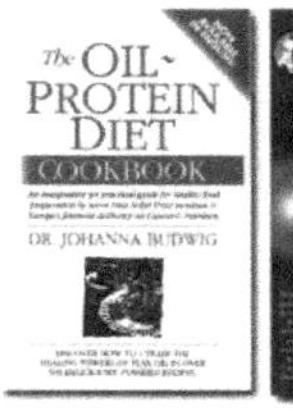

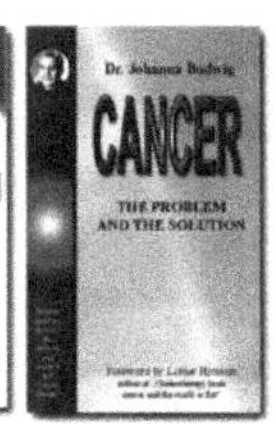

Delicious, delicate and descent way
To
Defeat dreadful disease the Cancer

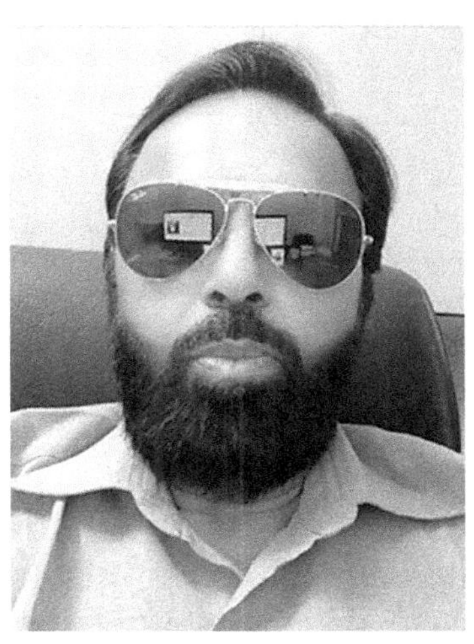

Written by
Dr. O.P.Verma
M.B.B.S., M.R.S.H. (London)
President, Flax Awareness Society
7-B-43, Mahaveer Nagar III, Kota (Raj.)
http://Flaxindia.blogspot.in
http://budwig.in
+919460816360

For cancers in the **prostate** or in the **breast**, the tumor is often dissolved or eliminated within a few weeks. This aid is even possible after cytostatic treatment and in the presence of metastasis.

The effect of this oil-protein cure for **brain tumors** in the lateral ventricle of the brain is very surprising.

For **leukemia** the success with children is fast and clear. The nutrition-based cause is quite noticeable here. For older persons with leukemia and tumor in the spleen, success is not so fast, but it is clear.

Dr. Johanna Budwig
(From Cancer The Problem And The Solution)

Foreword by Lothar Hirneise

My Teacher - Dr. Johanna Budwig

It is a great pleasure for me to write this foreword. I really appreciate how much energy Dr. O.P.Verma invested in the last ten years to learn, to practice and to spread the brilliance of the oil-protein diet in India. I hope that most cancer patients will read this book and learn the basis of this great cancer therapy. This book will definitely add a new dimension in the Alternative Cancer Treatment scenario and will prove a new mile stone in the awareness of Budwig Protocol.

First time I heard of Dr. Johanna Budwig and the oil-protein diet was precisely in America, as Frank Wiewel, President of People Against Cancer, USA told me that he had been in contact with Dr. Budwig for several years. He advised me to visit Dr. Budwig because I lived only one hour by car away from her home in Germany. I then visited Dr. Budwig in the spring of 1998 for the first time and from the beginning it was an intense relationship that persisted for many years.

Over several years I was a close companion of this grand dame of Science and we drank a few glasses of champagne together and discussion only interrupted by her afternoon nap, which she always held, countless hours about nutrition, oncology, church and many medical things in general. I had for several years the great good fortune to learn the opinions of Dr. Budwig, from the first hand and I will be eternally grateful for her.

Dr. Budwig was never married, always lived for science and almost her entire life dealt with other scientists. This was certainly not a simple life, and because in the family circle she had nobody to talk to about her oil-protein diet, she sometimes was glad that she found in me someone she could talk to about her theories. Thus it came about that she suggested one day to write a book in which she could explain her theories again briefly and concisely. And so the Book was made: Cancer - The Problem And The Solution.

I often visited her in Dietersweiler to discuss various opinions and her physical and mental faculties at that time were incredible for a woman of nearly 90 years. I had the feeling that once again she really inspired to write a book and every time when I came to her, there were already numerous articles and books on one of her three desks, and she wanted to discuss them with me.

The content of our conversations of course was about fat and electrons. Furthermore she helped me to improve my analytical thinking and I am always grateful for her instructions and how to basically question everything positive analytically. The oil-protein diet is not just for me and not only for cancer patients, it was something very special. In the past 15 years, I convinced myself personally of the effectiveness of this diet and for me it is now the base of my 3E-program.

Lothar Hirneise

Founder and President
People against Cancer Germany
www.3e-centre.com
www.nexus-health.com
www.hirneise.com
www.nexus-book.com

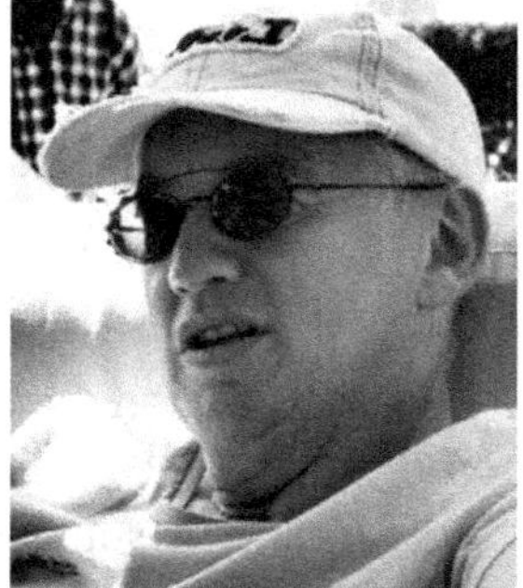

Table of Contents

Prime Cause of Cancer

We are fighting with cancer since the dawn of history. Every year we discover new diagnostic modalities, better radiotherapy techniques and lots of new chemotherapy drugs. But we have completely failed to defeat this disease called cancer. Think again, are we really going on the right path? Does conventional Medicine really targets upon the prime cause of cancer???

Otto Warburg – Biography

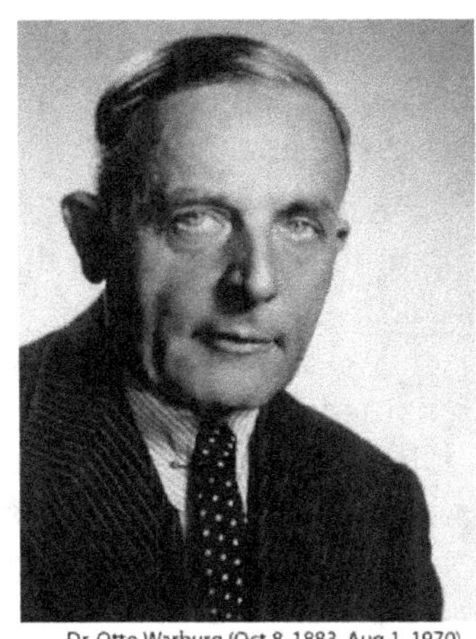

Dr. Otto Warburg (Oct 8, 1883 Aug 1, 1970)

Otto Heinrich Warburg (October 8, 1883 – August 1, 1970), son of physicist Emil Warburg, was a German physiologist, medical doctor and Nobel laureate. His mother was the daughter of a Protestant family of bankers and civil servants from Baden. Warburg studied chemistry under the great Emil Fischer, and earned his "Doctor of Chemistry" in Berlin in 1906. He then earned the degree of "Doctor of Medicine" in Heidelberg in 1911. Between 1908 and 1914, Warburg was affiliated with the Naples Marine Biological Station, in Naples, Italy, where he conducted research.

He served as an officer in the elite Uhlan (cavalry regiment) during the First World War, and was given the Iron Cross (1st Class) award for his bravery. Warburg is considered one of the 20th century's leading biochemists. Towards the end of the war, Albert Einstein, who had been a friend of Warburg's father Emil, wrote Warburg asking him to leave the army and return to academia, since it would be a tragedy for the world to lose his talents. Einstein and Warburg later became friends, and Einstein's work in physics had great influence on Otto's biochemical research.

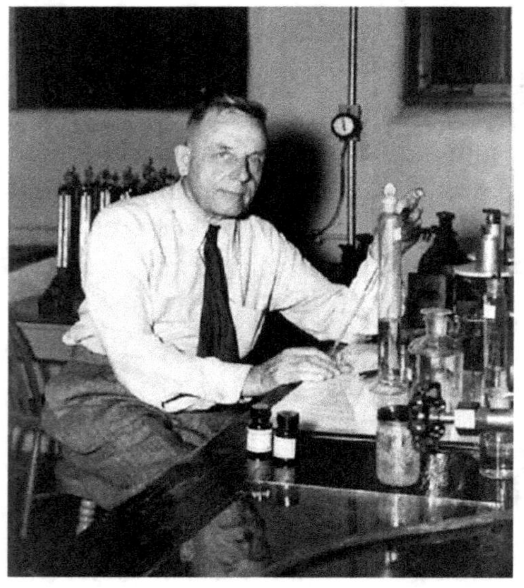

While working at the Marine Biological Station, Warburg performed research on oxygen consumption in sea urchin eggs after fertilization, and proved that upon fertilization, the rate of respiration increases by as much as six fold. His experiments also proved that iron is essential for the development of the larval stage.

In 1918, Warburg was appointed professor at the Kaiser Wilhelm Institute for Biology in Berlin-Dahlem. By 1931 he was promoted as director of the Kaiser Wilhelm Institute for Cell Physiology, which was later on, renamed the Max Planck Society. Warburg investigated the metabolism of tumors and the respiration of cells, particularly cancer cells, and in 1931 was awarded the Nobel Prize in Physiology for his "discovery of the nature and mode of action of the respiratory enzyme."

Nomination for a second Nobel Prize

In 1944, Warburg was nominated for a second Nobel Prize in Physiology by Albert Szent-Györgyi, for his work on nicotinamide, the mechanism and enzymes involved in fermentation, and the discovery of flavin (in yellow enzymes), but was prevented from receiving it by Adolf Hitler's regime.

Otto Warburg edited and had much of his original work published in The Metabolism of Tumors and wrote New Methods of Cell Physiology (1962). Otto Warburg was thrilled when Oxford University awarded him an honorary doctorate.

In his later years, Warburg was convinced that illness is resulted from pollution; this caused him to become a bit of a health advocate. He insisted on eating bread made from wheat grown organically on his farm. When he visited restaurants, he often made arrangements to pay 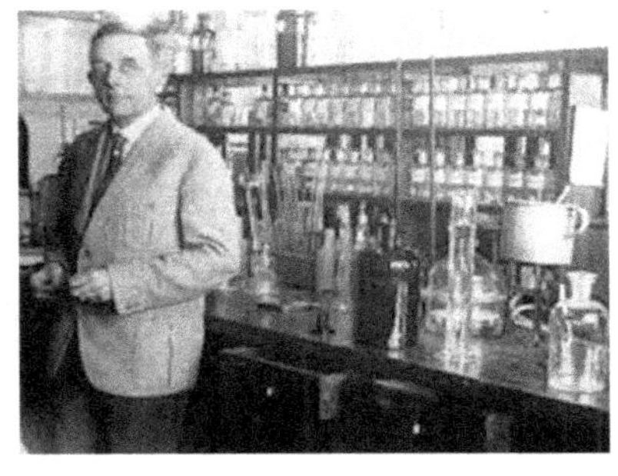 the full price for a cup of tea, but to only be served boiling water, from which he would make tea with a tea bag he had brought with him. He was also known to go to significant lengths to obtain organic butter, the quality of which he trusted.

The Otto Warburg Medal

The Otto Warburg Medal is intended to commemorate Warburg's outstanding achievements. It has been awarded by the German Society for Biochemistry and Molecular Biology since 1963. The prize honors and encourages pioneering achievements in fundamental biochemical and molecular biological research. The Otto Warburg Medal is regarded as the highest award for biochemists and molecular biologists in Germany.

Prime cause of Cancer

Warburg hypothesized that cancer growth is caused by tumor cells mainly generating energy (as e.g. adenosine triphosphate / ATP) by anaerobic breakdown of glucose (known as fermentation, or anaerobic respiration). This is in contrast to healthy cells, which mainly generate energy from oxidative breakdown of pyruvate. Pyruvate is an end product of glycolysis, and is oxidized within the mitochondria. Hence, and according to Warburg, cancer should be interpreted as a mitochondrial dysfunction.

In short, Warburg summarized that all normal cells absolutely require oxygen, but cancer cells can live without oxygen - a rule without exception. Deprive a cell 35% of its oxygen for 48 hours and it would become cancerous. **Dr. Otto Warburg clearly mentioned that the root cause of cancer is lack of oxygen in the cells.**

He also discovered that cancer cells are anaerobic (do not breathe oxygen), get the energy by fermenting glucose and produce levo-rotating lactic acid, and the body becomes acidic. Cancer cannot survive in the presence of high levels of oxygen, as found in an alkaline state.

He postulated that sulfur containing protein and some unknown fat is required to attract oxygen into the cell. This fat plays a major role in the respiration and functioning of Warburg respiratory enzyme. He thought it would be butyric acid and made experiment, but this attempt was a failure. For many decades scientists were trying to identify this unknown and mysterious fat but nobody succeeded (Otto Warburg, Wikipedia).

New Research supports Warburg's hypothesis

In 2006, a collaborative research team under the direction of Prof. Dr. Michael Ristow from the Universities of Jena and Potsdam was able to confirm the over 80 year old hypothesis of the Nobel Prize winner, Otto Warburg. Using the example of colon cancer in animal models, the team of scientists demonstrated the process of fermentation in tumor cells. The aerobic cellular respiration in these cancer cells could be restored again through treatment with a certain protein. The result showed that the animals tested had lost the ability to produce malignant tumors. This served as proof that the rate of tumor growth depends on certain metabolic processes and that these can be manipulated successfully.

US biologists, specifically a research team led by Michael and Thomas Seyfried Kiebish from Boston College, re-investigated the Warburg hypothesis in 2009. They concentrated intensely on the structure and function of the mitochondrial membrane in mice with different brain tumors. Mitochondria are cellular organelles called- in other words constituents of the cell- and the actual site of cellular respiration. In their observations, particular attention was given to a substance called cardiolipin- a phospholipid which stabilizes the mitochondrial membrane. There were significant differences in the membrane structure between healthy and diseased mice. The cardiolipins of the diseased mice were composed differently, resulting in a disruption of one of the most vital aspects of metabolism- namely electron transport- and thus to interfering with the entire energy production process. These results support the Warburg hypothesis.

Autobiography of Dr. Johanna Budwig

Birth of an angel

A lovely couple, Hermann Budwig and Elisabeth, lived in Essen town of Germany situated on the bank of river Ruhr. On the eve of 30th September, 1908 Elisabeth delivered a brilliant and lucky angel. Hermann and 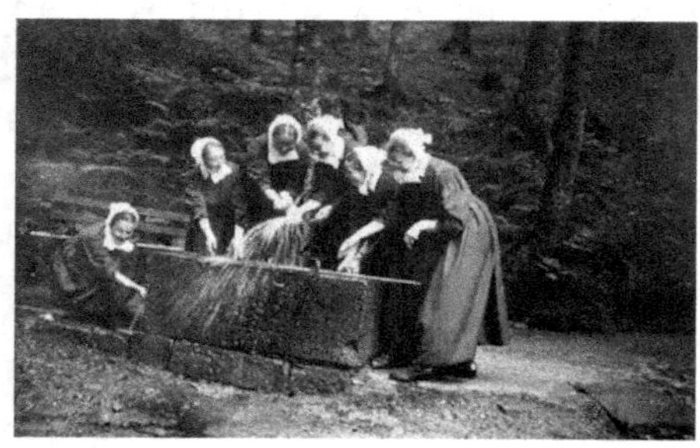 Elisabeth were very happy, and celebrating. They called her Johanna. In German, Johanna means a gift from God. In the family and neighborhood everybody was talking that Johanna is very lucky, she will study in a college and become a big doctor. Actually, 1908 was very fortunate and important year for the freedom of women in Germany. Government for the first time in history, changed laws, and allowed women to study in college and Universities. Also the German parliament passed a legislation to allow women to become members of political parties and prestigious clubs. Though women were given new rights and freedom, liberalization was slow and old values still persisted.

The tough life of a sage of science

Unluckily, Elisabeth died in 1920; family members thought that her father, being a poor loco mechanic, might not look after Johanna. So she was sent to an orphanage. This was a great shock for the little Johanna, but it had one positive side also. Education up to higher level was totally free for orphans.

In 1926, Germany was slowly recovering from the after effects of the First World War. Economic conditions were improving. Scholars and scientists were developing new technologies in every field. One third of all Nobel Prizes were being given to German academics.

Deaconess at Kaiserswerth

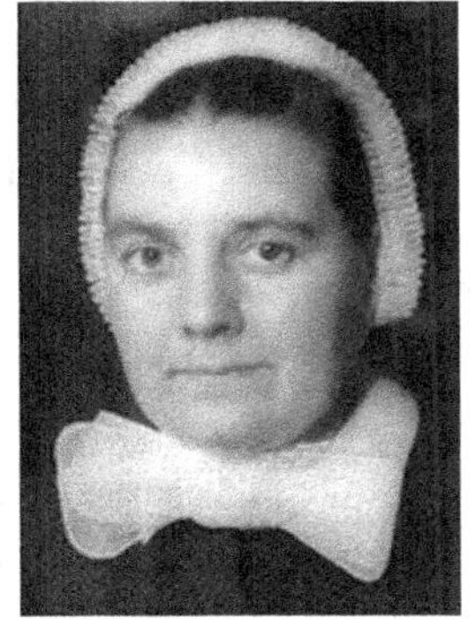

Johanna was very intelligent and sharp in studies from the beginning. In order to achieve good future, she decided to join the renowned Deaconess's Institute of Kaiserswerth in 1925. Theodor Fliedner, a pastor, founded Kaiserswerth Institute for welfare of unmarried mothers, prisoners, patients, orphans and poor children in 1836. In the beginning a Hospital and a Nursing School was established. This school was very famous Nursing School of that time. Florence Nightingale, known as mother of modern nursing, also studied in this Deaconess School in 1850. Intelligent Johanna easily got admission in this Institute. She was made a "deaconess" on March 30, 1932. This was the most appropriate place for her. There was a 1000 bedded hospital, pharmacy and a boarding school. She decided to study pharmacy.

After completing preliminary education in Kaiserswerth, she joined Münster University for further studies. Her analytical thinking and precise knowledge was noticed by her Professor Dr Hans Paul Kaufmann. He always encouraged and helped her. Here she passed state examination in pharmacy and was rewarded distinction in chemistry in 1936. Then she continued further education in physics, and received the title "Doctor of Science" at the University of Münster in 1938. On August 1, 1939, she was appointed as in-charge of pharmacy at the Military Hospital in Kaiserswerth.

Next month, Hitler's military forces attacked Poland. During war time, brave Johanna was busy in organizing and expanding the pharmacy. The war was not an easy time. There were two thousand people living in Kaiserswerth. Johanna was responsible for ensuring that there were enough medicines in this time of rationing and a thriving black market. She was well prepared and ready to fulfill any emergency demand for her patients. Many of her fellow deaconesses were often jealous and not co-operating but she continued evolving her professional skills. She was strong and was confronting every opponent (Dr. Johanna Budwig Stiftung).

Dr Budwig's scientific thinking, work and career

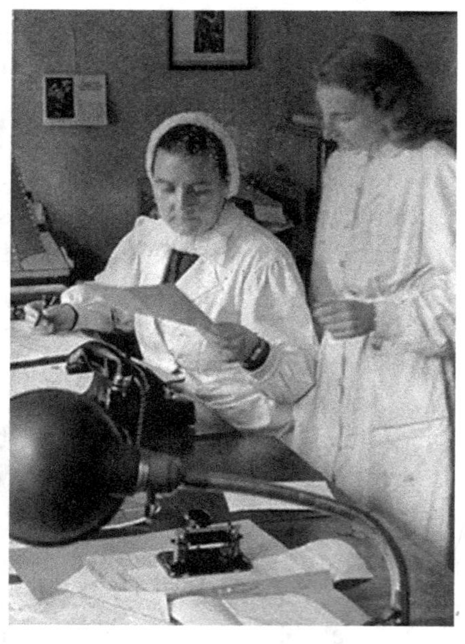

After Second World War, Johanna left Kaiserswerth in 1949. Soon Prof. Kaufmann came to know that she had left Kaiserswerth. He immediately met and persuaded her to work with him in Münster University, as he was always impressed from her talent. He converted the basement of his house into a laboratory and arranged all facilities for her research. He was famous as Fat Pope in the whole Europe.

On Prof. Kaufmann's recommendation, Johanna was appointed as the chief expert for drugs and fats at the Federal Institute for Fats Research, Germany. This was the country's largest office issuing the approval of new drugs used for cancer. Many applications had been submitted to her for approval. These were the medications for cancer therapy with the sulfhydryl group (sulfur-containing protein compounds). Everywhere she saw that fats played a role in cellular respiration, also in expert reports provided by well-known professors like Prof. Nonnenbruch. Unfortunately, fats could only be detected in the late stage, and there were no method to distinguish between fats chemically.

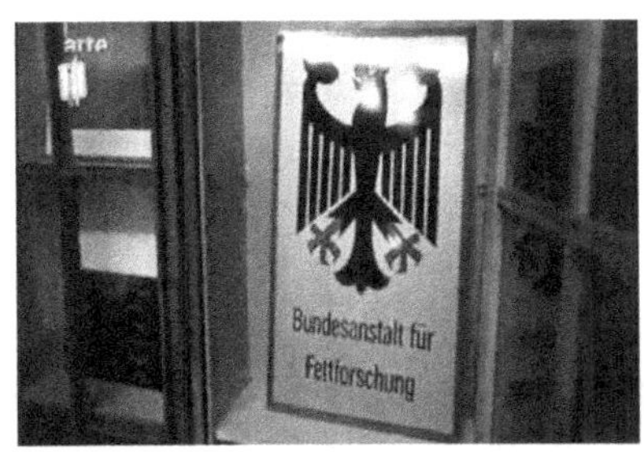

By this time, she developed paper chromatography. With this technique for first time she was able to detect fatty acids and lipoproteins directly even in 0.1 ml of blood. She used Co60 isotopes successfully to produce the first differential reaction for fatty acids, and produced the first direct iodine value via radioiodine. She also developed control of atmosphere in a closed system by using gas systems which act as antioxidants. She further developed Coloring methods, separating effects of fats and fatty acids. She too studied their behavior in blue and red light with fluorescent dyes.

Using rhodamine red dye, she studied the electrical behavior of the unsaturated fatty acids with their "halo". With this technique she could prove that electron rich highly unsaturated Linoleic and Linolenic fatty acids (Flax oil being the richest source) were the mysterious and undiscovered decisive fats required to attract oxygen into the cells, which Otto Warburg could not find. She studied the electromagnetic function of pi-electrons of the linolenic acid in the cell membranes, for nerve function, secretions, mitosis, as well as cell division. She also examined the synergism of the sulfur containing protein with the pi-electrons of the highly unsaturated fatty acids and their significance for the formation of the hydrogen bridge between fat and protein, which represent "the only path" for fast and focused Transport of electrons during respiration. This research was extensively published in 1950 in Neue Wege in der Fettforschung (New Directions in Fat Research) and other publications.

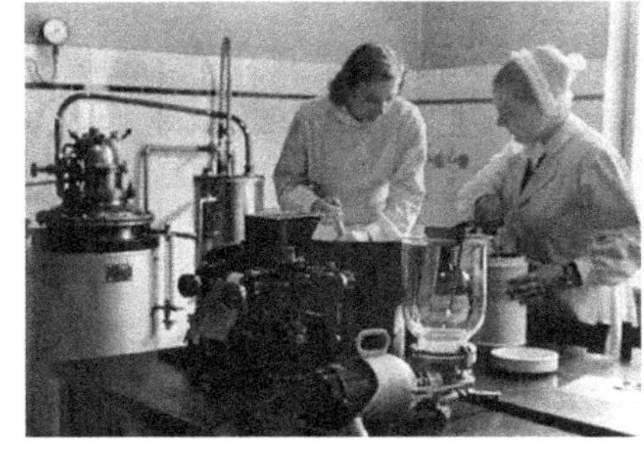

This immediately caused an excitement and turmoil in the scientific community. Everybody thought that it would open new doors in Cancer research. She also proved that hydrogenated fats and refined oils including all Trans-fatty acids were not having vital electrons and were respiratory poisons.

During her research, she found that the blood of seriously ill cancer patients had deficiency of unsaturated essential fats (Linoleic and Linolenic fatty acids), lipoproteins, phosphatides, and hemoglobin. She also had noticed that cancer 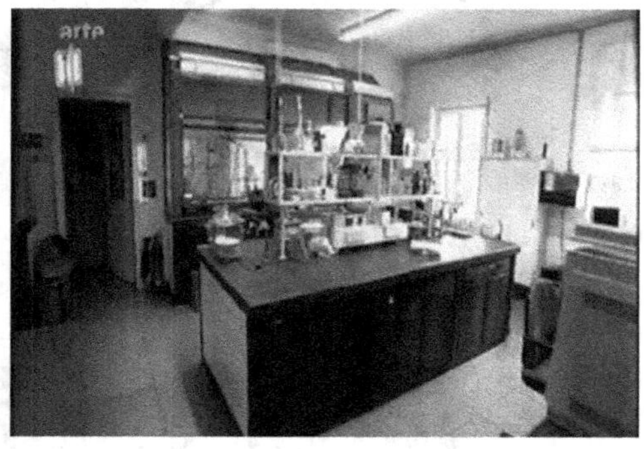 patients had a strange greenish-yellow substance in their blood which is not present in the blood of healthy people (Budwig, Cancer The Problem And The Solution).

She wanted to develop a healing program for cancer. So she enrolled over 642 cancer patients from four hospitals in Münster. She gave Flax oil and Cottage Cheeseto these patients. After just three months, patients began to improve in health and strength, the yellow green substance in their blood began to disappear, tumors gradually receded and at the same time the nutrients began to rise.

This way she developed a simple cure for cancer, based on the consumption of Flax oil with low fat Quark or cottage cheese, raw organic diet, mild exercise, Flax oil massage and the healing powers of the sun. It was a great victory and the first milestone in the battle against cancer. She treated approx. 2500 cancer patients during last few decades. Prof. Halme of surgery clinic in Helsinki used to keep records of her patients. According to him her success was over 90%, and this was achieved in cases, which were rejected by Allopathic doctors.

Dr. Budwig was a courageous scientist. She **loudly and convincingly argued that consumption of highly processed foods, particularly edible oils and margarines, which block the oxidation processes in the cells, are responsible for the development of cancer and other degenerative diseases.** She met with great resistance from food industry giants, who were doing everything to prevent the spread of her sensational discovery. In 1952, under the influence of strong pressure from this lobby, she lost her job and was barred from the research work.

Joins Medical School at Göttingen

Opponents of Dr. Johanna blamed her that she should not treat cancer patients because she doesn't have a doctor's degree. She felt this and eventually joined medical school in Göttingen in

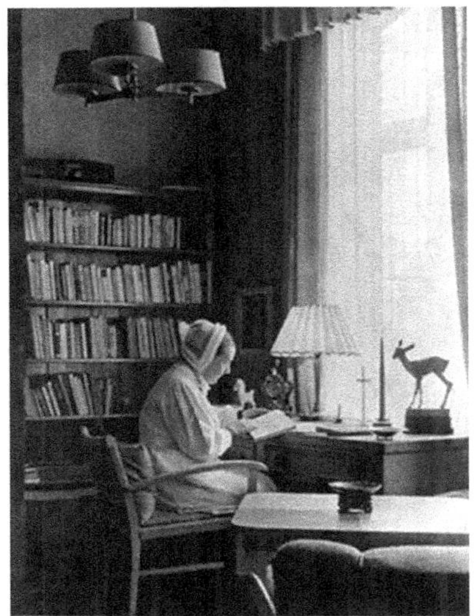

1955. Budwig was 47 years old at that time. She also continued her research work along with her studies. *Budwig successfully treated Prof. Martius's wife, who suffered from Breast Cancer*

One night a woman came with her small child whose arm was supposed to be amputated due to a tumor. She treated her and soon the amputation surgery was dismissed, and the child quickly did very well.

A Swiss woman came to her clinic in Göttingen. She suffered from Colon Cancer with metastasis and intestinal obstruction. Several doctors examined her, and was to be operated on Christmas Eve. On Budwig's request, she was treated by her protocol. The tumor of the colon quickly subsided. Seven weeks later, she was discharged without any detectable tumor. It is interesting that the Swiss custom officer was not ready to believe that the submitted passport belonged to same lady. Her look was so much changed! At home her daughter welcomed saying: "You look healthy, younger and more beautiful (from her book The Death of the Tumor – Vol. II).

After this, University allowed her to treat cancer patients with her oil-protein diet. She was getting miraculous results. University professors were excited with the results, but wanted that she should also include chemo and radiotherapy. She was rigid and didn't want to compromise. So she had differences and conflicts with her professors and ultimately left Göttingen (Budwig, Cancer The Problem And The Solution).

Last Destination - Dietersweiler-Freudenstadt

Eventually, she shifted to Dietersweiler-Freudenstadt, where she lived till her death. There she completed Ph.D. in Naturopathy so that she could legally treat cancer patients. She continued treating her patients in Freudenstadt. In 1968 she created unique Eldi oils for massage and enema, called Electron Differential Oils after performing precise spectroscopic measurements of the light absorption in different oils. *US pain institute has written somewhere: "What this crazy woman does with her ELDI oils, none of us manages to do via pain killers."*

Budwig conducted more than 200 lectures worldwide. Dr. Budwig was popular in the U.S. as FLAX SEED lady from Freudenstadt. She delivered her last public Lecture in Freudenstadt on March 3, 1999. On November 28, 2002, she fell down in her bathroom and got a fracture in right femur neck. She was admitted in a nursing home and ultimately died on May 19, 2003.

Below are pictures are of the **Federal Institute for Fat Research in Germany** where Dr. Budwig worked at.

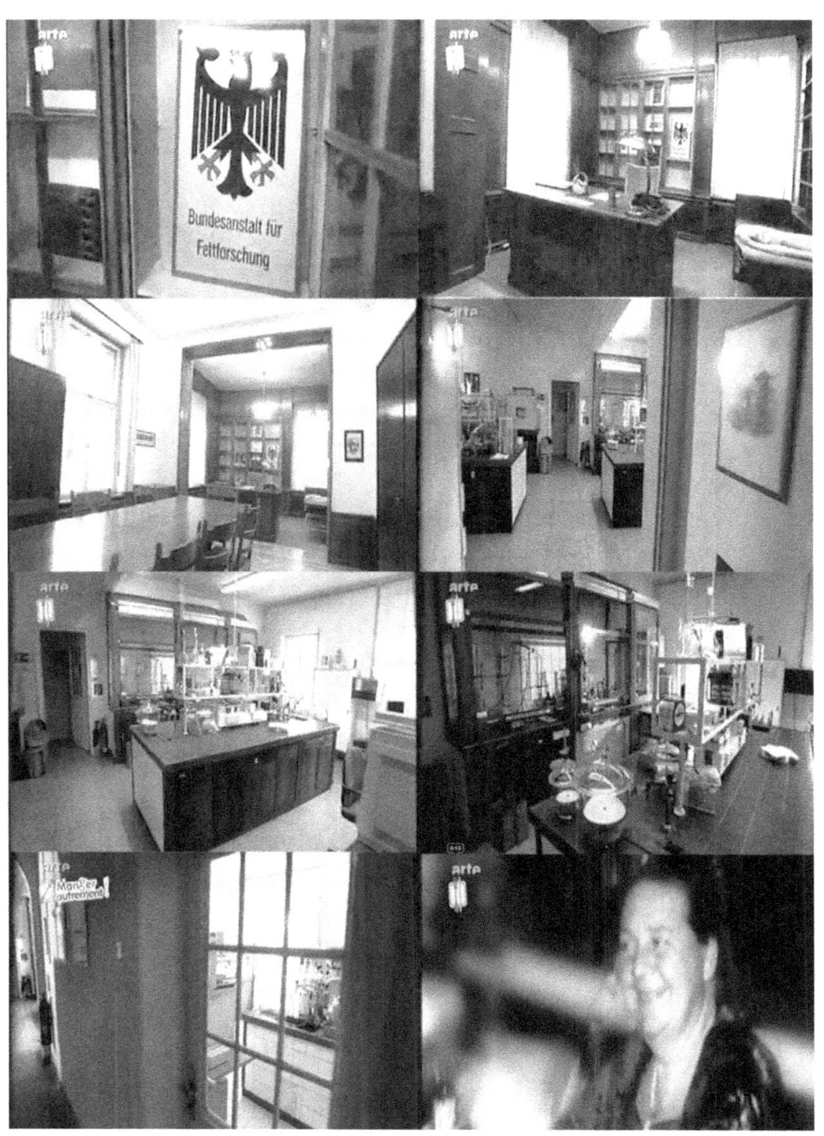

Dr. Johanna Budwig's Works in English

- Flax Oil As A True Aid Against Arthritis, Heart Infarction, Cancer, And Other Diseases by Dr. Johanna Budwig
- The Oil-Protein Diet Cookbook by Dr. Johanna Budwig
- Cancer - The Problem and The Solution by Dr Johanna Budwig

Dr. Johanna Budwig's books in German

- Krebs - Das Problem und die LösungKrebs - by Johanna Budwig
- Öl-Eiweiß-KostÖl-Eiweiß-Kost [The Oil-Protein Diet Cookbook] by Johanna Budwig
- Kosmische Kräfte gegen KrebsKosmische Kräfte gegen Krebs [Cosmic Forces Against Cancer] by Johanna Budwig. Hyperion-Verlag, Germany (1966)
- Krebs, ein FettproblemKrebs, ein Fettproblem. Richtige Wahl und Verwendung der Fette [Cancer - A Fats Problem, on the right choice and use of fats] by Johanna Budwig, Hyperion, Freiburg, Germany (1967)
- Fette als wahre Hilfe gegen Arteriosklerose, Herzinfarkt, Krebs u. a.Fette als wahre Hilfe gegen Arteriosklerose, Herzinfarkt, Krebs u. a. Drei Vorträge. [published in English as FlaxOil As A True Aid Against Arthritis, Heart Infarction, Cancer, And Other Diseases. Three Lectures] by Johanna Budwig, Hyperion, Frbg. Germany (1972)
- Die elementare Funktion der Atmung in ihrer Beziehung zu autoxydablen Nahrungsstoffen Die elementare Funktion der Atmung in ihrer Beziehung zu autoxydablen Nahrungsstoffen [The Elementary Function of Respiration in its Relationship to Autoxydable Foodstuffs] by Johanna Budwig
- Das Fettsyndrom Das Fettsyndrom [The Fat Syndrome] by Johanna Budwig Hyperion, Frbg., Germany (1972)

- Die elementare Funktion der Atmung in ihrer Beziehung zu autoxydablen NahrungsstoffenFettfibel by Budwig
- Der Tod des Tumors, Bd. I, by Johanna Budwig 1977
- Die elementare Funktion der Atmung in ihrer Beziehung zu autoxydablen Nahrungsstoffen Der Tod des Tumors, Bd. II by Johanna Budwig 1977
- Die elementare Funktion der Atmung in ihrer Beziehung zu autoxydablen Nahrungsstoffen Laserstrahlen gegen Krebs by Johanna Budwig Hyperion, Frbg., Germany (1968)
- Die elementare Funktion der Atmung in ihrer Beziehung zu autoxydablen Nahrungsstoffen Fotoelemente des Lebens by Johanna Budwig Resch Verlag, Innsbruck (1979)
- Die elementare Funktion der Atmung in ihrer Beziehung zu autoxydablen Nahrungsstoffen Inaugural Disputation by Johanna Budwig (November 1979)
- "Dieses Manuskript mit Einleitung liegt dem Karolinska Medico Kirurgiska Institut Stockholm vor, in englischer Sprache. Der Nobelpreis für Medizin wurde für die Autorin vorgeschlagen von mehreren Vertretern der Medizin aus dem In- und Auslande."
- Die elementare Funktion der Atmung in ihrer Beziehung zu autoxydablen Nahrungsstoffen Mensch sein. Atmung, Immunabwehr im Würgegriff by Johanna Budwig (1986/87)

Lothar Herniece's new books in English

- Oil-Protein Diet (New book)
- Oil-Protein Cookbook (New Edition)
- Cancer The Problem And The Solution (New Edition)
- Chemotherapy Heals Cancer And World Is Flat

(These books are available at http://www.hirneise.com/page-8/page-19/)

Budwig Protocol

The Budwig Protocol is one of the most widely followed alternative treatments for cancer and other diseases. The diet seems simple, but foods are powerful and can heal a person.

Transition Diet

The Transition diet is especially recommended for patients of liver, pancreatic or gall bladder cancers. The basic principle is that for 3 days nothing is eaten and drunk except the following written and at least three times daily warm tea (herbal teas from peppermint, rose hip, mallow or green tea) is drunk. Dr Budwig has recommended variant 1 for patients with a relatively good energy state, and variant 2 and 3 mainly for seriously ill patients.

Variant 1

Variant 1 for three days, 250 g of linomel or alternatively freshly crushed Flax seed is eaten together with the following:

- Freshly pressed fruit juices without added sugar.
- Freshly pressed vegetable juices such as carrot, celery juice, red beetroots and apple juice.
- Chinese tea and black tea are allowed in the morning
- Honey for sweetening is allowed. Just as grape juice for drinking and as a sweetener. Energetically weak patients can also consume sparkling wine and linomel.

Variant 2

For three days, oat meal cereal very hour with linomel is eaten daily with the following juices:

- Freshly pressed fruit juices or freshly pressed vegetable juices such as carrot, celery juice, beetroot and apple juice.
- Chinese tea and black tea are allowed in the morning.

- Honey for sweetening is allowed. Just as grape juice for drinking and as a sweetener.
- Energetically weak patients can also consume sparkling wine and linomel.

Variant 3

For three days, oatmeal soup with linomel is given three times a day together with the following juices:

- Freshly pressed fruit juices or fruit juices without added sugar.
- Freshly pressed vegetable juices such as carrot, celery juice, beetroot and apple juice.
- Chinese tea and black tea are allowed in the morning.
- Honey for sweetening is allowed. Just as grape juice for drinking and as a sweetener.
- Energetically weak patients can also consume sparkling wine and linomel.

It is often experienced frequently that patients mixed all three variants and "nevertheless" had good results. So better you to stick to one variant. (Budwig – Cancer The Problem And The Solution 2005: p.36).

Budwig Diet

The Budwig Protocol is necessary for many diseases from cancer to type 2 diabetes and heart disease to autoimmune diseases, etc. Its purpose is to energize the cells by restoring the natural electrical potential in the cell. Many human diseases are caused by "sick cells" which have lost their normal electrical potential; generally via a lower ATP energy in the cell's mitochondria.

6:00 AM – Sauerkraut juice

A glass of sauerkraut juice consumed before breakfast every morning. It is rich in vitamins including C, enzymes and helps develop the health-promoting gut flora. Sauerkraut is cabbage that has been pickled by natural fermentation, mainly with lactobacillus bacteria. It is slightly salty, sharp and sour. Well made, it is much nicer than it sounds. You may also consume another glass of sauerkraut juice later in the day.

It interesting that sauerkraut contains right rotating lactic acids and is highly alkaline and neutralizes levo-rotating lactic acids and makes our body alkaline. That is why Marcus Porcius Cato the Elder issued a statement - Carcinomas are incurable except with the treatment with Sauerkraut.

8:00 AM Breakfast

Green or herbal tea

Start breakfast with a cup of warm herbal or green tea. Sweeten with only natural honey. You can add lemon or grape juice. Patient should take such a tea before or with Linomel Muesli. You may consume 4-5 such teas in a day.

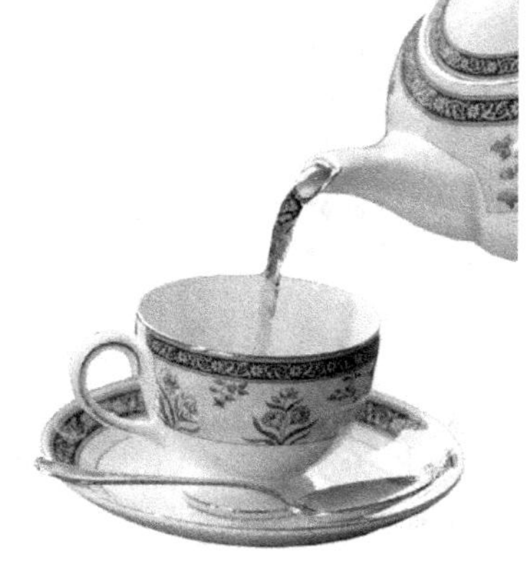

Linomel Muesli or Oil-Protein Muesli

This should be made fresh and consumed within 15 minutes. It is full of high energy pi-electrons, attract oxygen in the cells

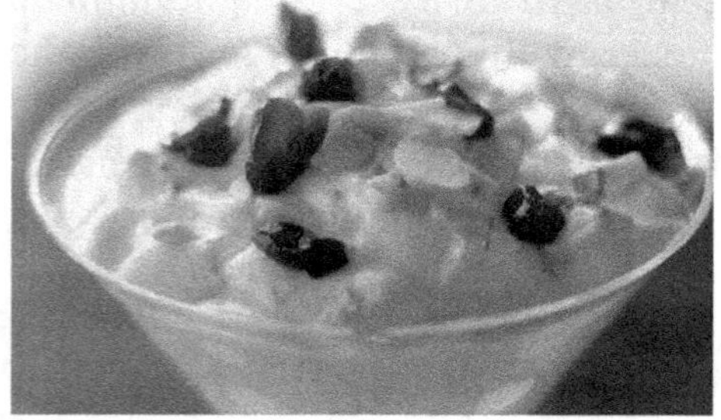

and capable of healing cell membranes. It is full of energy-rich omega-3 fats, has power to attract healing photons from sun through resonance. As "Om" is divine word and synonym of God in India. According to Hindu Mythology, the whole universe is located inside "Om", so the name Omkhand has been given to this wonderful recipe in Hindi.

Ingredients

- 3 Tbsp cold pressed organic Flax seed oil (FO)
- 100-125gm (6 Tbsp) Quark or Cottage Cheese(CC)
- 2 Tbsp freshly ground Flax seeds
- 2 Tbsp milk
- 1 cup fruits
- ¼ cup dried nuts
- Natural honey
- Flavorings – lemon, apple cider vinegar, cinnamon, pure cacao, natural vanilla, shredded coconut etc.

Recipe

Place 2 tablespoons Linomel or freshly ground Flax seeds in a small bowl. It is covered with raw, crushed or diced seasonal fruits depending on the season. Pour some orange or grape juice over this. Linomel^{Tm} is a brand name and originally created and patented by Budwig. It is a cereal made from cracked Flax Seed, a small amount of honey and a little milk powder.

Then the Quark-Flax seed oil cream is prepared in as follows: First add Flax seed oil, milk and honey and blend briefly with a hand-held immersion electric blender, then gradually add the Quark in smaller portions. Blend till oil and Quark is thoroughly mixed with no separated oil. Then it is seasoned differently everyday with different flavorings such as vanilla, cinnamon or various fruits such as banana, apple, lemon, orange juice, or berries.

Use various fruits such as fresh berries, apple, cherry, orange, banana, papaya, grapes etc. Add other fresh fruit if you like, totaling 1/2 to 1 cup of fruit. Budwig specially advised to use berries like strawberry, blueberry, raspberry, cheery

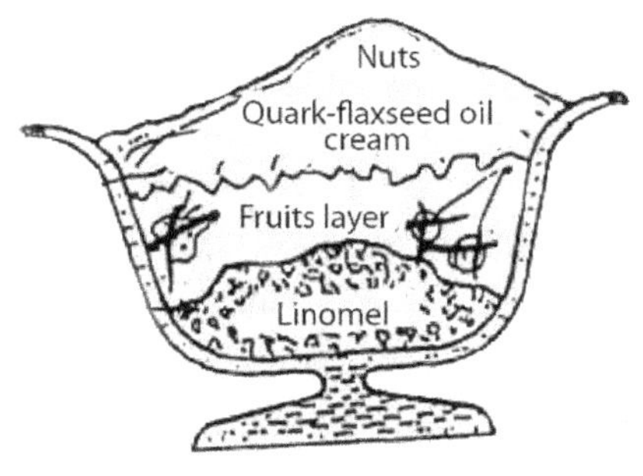

19

etc. because berries have ellagic acids which are strong cancer fighters.

Add organic raw nuts such as walnuts, almonds, raisins or Brazil nuts. They have sulfurated proteins, omega-3 fats and vitamins. Brazil nut is especially important because a single nut provides you with all of the selenium you need for the day. Selenium is very important to boost immune power. Peanuts are prohibited.

For variety and flavor, try natural vanilla, cinnamon, lemon juice, pure cocoa or shredded coconut.

Once blended in Budwig Cream, Quark and Flax seed oil form a new substance called lipoprotein. Lipoprotein is a water soluble complex. The Quark is rich in the sulfur-containing amino acids, methionine and cysteine. These positively charged amino acids attract the negatively charged electron clouds in fatty acid chains and exhibit a stabilizing effect on the highly unsaturated, otherwise easily oxidized fats. Thus, the amino acids protect the polyunsaturated fatty acids from the Flax seed oil against oxidation which, as a result, are able to enter the human body unchanged and with their full energy potential. The result: they are much more valuable to cells and their membranes. Consequently, one could say that Quark excels as a protector for the polyunsaturated fatty acids.

Sulfur-rich amino acids play a wealth of roles in many vital functions in our bodies. In combination with polyunsaturated fatty acids, they are important partners in regulating the uptake of oxygen and its utilization by the cell. They therefore contribute significantly to a strong immune system, healthy metabolism, and mental vitality. For many generations, people have been getting their omega-3 fatty acids from fish, vegetables, nuts, and seeds. Our health literally depends on the regular consumption of the essential omega-3 and omega-6 fatty acids, alpha-linolenic acid (ALA) and linoleic acid (LA). Our bodies require these fatty acids in order to synthesize their cell membranes as well as for a variety of metabolic processes and heal the cancer and other diseases.

Tips for making the Budwig Mixture

- Follow directions properly! It is important to add things to the mixture in the right order. If you mix them in the wrong order you may lose a lot of the opportunity to convert the oil-soluble omega-3 into water soluble-omega-3.
- Keep the Flax seed oil refrigerated.
- Immersion blender is a must.
- The mixture can be flavored differently every day by adding nuts and fruits preferably organic such as pecans, almonds or walnuts (not peanuts), banana, organic cocoa, shredded coconut, pineapple (fresh) blueberries, raspberries, cinnamon, vanilla or (freshly) squeezed fruit juice.
- Consume immediately for best results.

10 AM Vegetable juice

Freshly squeezed vegetable juice from carrots, beets, celery, tomato, and radish, lemon as well as green vegetables - stinging nettle, lettuce or spinach. Apple is added to sweeten and enhance the taste. Carrot & beet juices are especially helpful to the liver and have strong cancer fighting properties. Vary vegetables. Some tasty and nutritious combinations are beet and apple juice, carrot and apple, carrot and beet, asparagus and apple, celery and apple, celery and carrot. Beet juice should not be taken alone. If taken alone it may cause red or pink urine (beeturia).

She also frequently recommended the following juices:

1. Nettle juice - Especially in the spring, Dr Budwig recommended to puree nettles with water and a lemon.

2. Radish juice - For this, a radish is first crushed and then thrown together with a lemon into the juicer. This juice is by the way durable for several days and Dr Budwig has sometimes recommended her patients to drink a small quantity of them every day.

3. Coltsfoot juice - For this juice, with the exception of the harder old rootstock, the entire remaining underground shoot is mixed with a few flowers and some milk and honey.

4. Horseradish juice - Mix 3-5 cm horseradish together with an apple and (raw) milk. Depending on the quantity of milk you can change the taste. Dr Budwig recommended this juice above all to workmen and to stimulate the appetite. Freshly pressed means, by the way, that you drink the juice within 5 minutes after pressing. In some cases, Dr Budwig prescribed a second juice 30 to 60 minutes later.

12:15 PM Lunch

Salad Platter: Salad plate with homemade cottage cheese-Flax seed mayonnaise. As salad also use: dandelion, cress, celery, tomato, cucumber, lettuce, radish, cabbage, broccoli, green horseradish and pepper.

Delicious mayo salad dressing can be prepared by mixing together 2 Tbsp (30 ml) Flax Oil, 2 Tbsp (30 ml) milk, and 2 Tbsp (30 ml) cottage cheese. Then add 2 tablespoons (30 ml) of Lemon juice (or Apple Cider Vinegar) and add 1 teaspoon (2.5 g) Mustard powder plus some herbs of your choice. Other alternative dressing can be made by mixing Flax Oil, lemon juice, Mustard and some herbs (Budwig, The Oil-Protein Diet Cookbook, 1994).

Main Course: Vegetables cooked in water, then flavored with Oleolox and herbs possibly with oatmeal, soy sauce, curry etc. Vegetable broth flavored with a little Oleolox and yeast flakes. As side dish for the

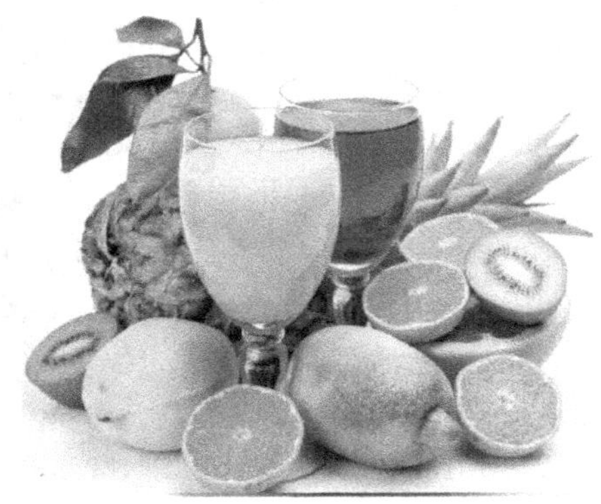

vegetables: buckwheat, brown rice, millet or potatoes can be used. One or two slices of Ezekiel bread can be taken. Use lot of dried fruits in the main meal also.

Lunch Dessert: Cottage cheese/ Flax oil mixture served as a dessert, prepared with dry fruits and fruits such as apple, or poured over a fruit salad. You already know how to prepare it perfectly. You will find wonderful recipes for a delicious dessert in the Oil-Protein cookbook by Budwig. Please note that the dessert is **"a must"** and should definitely be eaten. So keep your main course light so you may enjoy the dessert happily.

The form of preparation as "fruit foam," "Linovita" or "red coat in the snow" (in Oil-Protein cookbook) is always welcoming for the healthy and the sick. In all the gimmicks in the preparation of the delicious desserts, one should be aware: Quark and Flaxseed give the patient immense power within a short space of time. Always fresh and beautiful, always freshly interesting, this important food for life should be for the sick and for the whole family.

3 PM Fruit juices

In the afternoon, Dr Budwig recommended different kinds of fruit juices e.g. apples, grapes, cherries, pineapples, papaya, or apricot, sparkling wine or wine - with or without Flaxseeds or with or without a few drops Flaxseed oil.

3:30 PM Enzyme Juice

Budwig preferred papaya juice and recommended her patients to drink at least every 2 days a glass of papaya juice. The main reason for this was definitely the protein splitting enzyme papain.

6 PM Dinner

The evening meal should be light and served early, around 6 p.m. A warm meal may be prepared using brown rice, buckwheat or oat meal. Never consume corn or soy beans. Dishes made with buckwheat grouts are most easily tolerated and nourishing. Use only honey to sweeten. Soup or more solid dishes can be combined with a tasty sauce according to preference. Use OLEOLOX liberally also to sweet sauces and soups, making them nourishing and a richer source of energy.

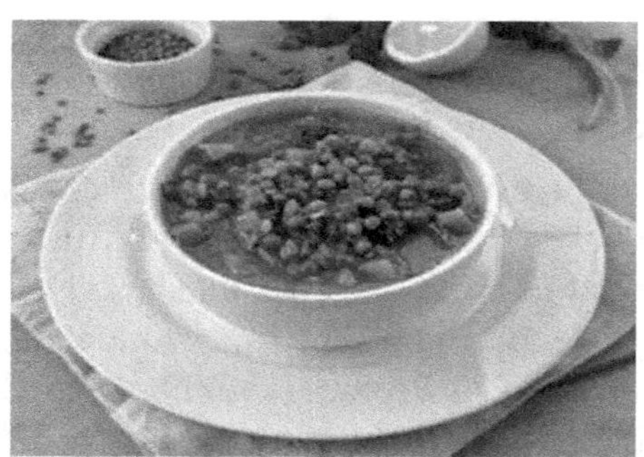

8:30 PM

A glass of organic red wine may be consumed. All things are a matter of correct dosage. This glass of red wine is not a "must" program. In fact, seriously ill patients having pain and discomfort just starting on the oil-protein diet, it is recommended to serve a glass of red wine mixed with freshly ground Flax seeds to tide them over while going off pain killers (Budwig, Cancer The Problem And The Solution).

METRIC CONVERSION TABLE	
10 g = 0.35 oz	5 cc = 1 teaspoon
100 g = 3.5 oz	15 cc = 1 tablespoon
150 g = 5.25 oz	30 cc = 1 ounce
250 g = 8.8 oz	250 cc = 1 cup
454 g = 1 lb	960 cc = 1 qt
Oz = ounce lb = pound qt = quart Tsp = teaspoon Tbsp = tablespoon	

Precautions

Drink filtered water - Use RO (Reverse Osmosis)water for drinking, cooking and enemas.

Eat Organic Diet - Always try to eat organic food.

Dental Care –

Mercury is a Carcinogenic as well as a Poison! The root canals of dead teeth are full of bacteria that attack the liver and lymphatic system. From Amalgam fillings the mercury slowly leaks out of the filings. The ADA cleverly defends the use of amalgam in spite of the fact that there is sufficient evidence that patients with many severe problems, including psychotic episodes and fatal allergic reactions, were just cured by removing the amalgam. It is advisable to rather have a ceramic filling than be slowly poisoned by mercury. Even gold filling is dangerous; it acts as battery producing electrical current. Be informed that the effect of drugs, including poison, is dose dependant and cumulative.

Fluoride is not only toxic but it is also carcinogenic. Fluoride has never been proven to prevent tooth decay. It has been outlawed in many countries or groups of countries because the evidence is overwhelming that fluoride causes premature aging, so drink bottled water and use fluoride-free toothpaste (American Cancer Institute - 1963).

I highly recommend helping you avoid fillings in the first place. Holistic dentist recommend 3% H_2O_2 as a gargle or rinse, or making a paste using baking soda. H_2O_2 usage three times a day is advised. It is great for cleaning dentures, too.

Frying and deep frying - Frying and deep frying is not allowed to cook patient's food. Never heat any oil in the kitchen. By heating oils the wealth of high energy electrons is destroyed and Tran's fats and dangerous toxic chemicals such as acrylamides are

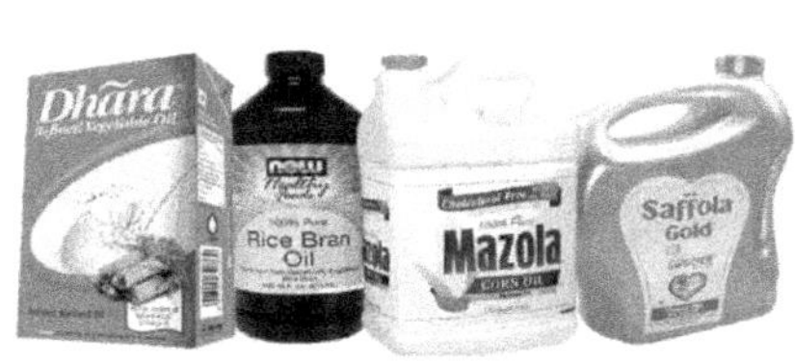

formed in the oil. Boiling and steaming are good practices. You can fry vegetables etc. in water and add oleolox before serving. Water is the safest medium for frying, says Lothar Hirneise.

Chemo and Radio -

Chemotherapy is aimed at destruction of the tumor, and it destroys many living cells, and the entire person. Anything that disturbs growth is fatal because growth is an elementary function of life. We cannot achieve something good with bad tools.

Dr. Budwig rejects Chemo and Radiation Therapy. Budwig used to say with full confidence and clarity, "My 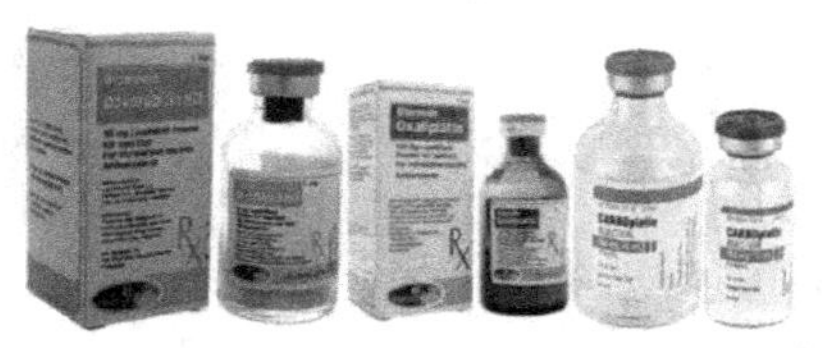 treatment targets on the real cause of cancer; it fills cancer cells with high energy pi-electrons and attracts oxygen into the cells. And cancer cells start to breathe and produce vital energy."

Man-made Supplements - With this treatment man-made antioxidants, synthetic vitamins and pain killers should not be given. The dose of anticoagulants and aspirin should be adjusted by your doctor. Dr. Budwig favors natural, herbal and homeopathy instead of man-made and synthetic supplements, vitamins and pain killers (Budwig, Cancer The Problem And The Solution).

Prohibitions of Budwig Protocol

In this protocol there are certain restrictions. They are as important as the diet itself. It is very difficult to defeat the cancer without strictly following these rules.

Sugar is strictly forbidden

Sugar, Jiggery, molasses, maple syrup and artificial sweeteners like xylitol, aspartame are not permitted. You can use only natural honey, Stevie and fruit juices – all off course unprocessed.

Avoid meats, eggs and fish

Meat, fish, poultry, eggs, and butter are never allowed. Preserved meat is like a poison. It is highly processed and treated with dangerous antibiotics, preservatives and nitrates.

Stop using Hydrogenated Fat and Refined oil

You can never eat pizza, burger, fast food, fried food, biscuits etc. as they all are made by hydrogenated margarine and shortenings. Hydrogenation is a very dangerous process, used to increase shelf life of fats. In this process (oil is heated at very high temperature and hydrogen is passed through oils in presence of nickel) killing Trans fats are formed, high energy live and vital electrons are destroyed and nutrients are damaged. Hydrogenated Fats is just a dead, nutrition-less and cancer causing liquid plastic. Budwig always preached against these damaging fats. She has allowed low fat cheese, oleolox and coconut oil.

Preservatives and Processed Food

You should not eat Potato chips, soft drinks etc. which are full of preservatives. Never consume highly processed food e.g. ready to eat packed foods, pasta, pastries, bread and soy products, tofu etc. However good quality soy souse is permitted.

Microwave, Teflon, Aluminum and Plastic

Never cook in microwave oven. Food cooked in microwave become toxic and deformed. Also don't use aluminum, plastic, Teflon coated cookware and aluminum foils. Use stainless steel, iron, china clay or glass utensils instead.

Chemicals and pesticides are not allowed

Avoid pesticides and chemicals, even those in household products & cosmetics. Stay away from mosquito repellants, sun screen lotions and sun glasses.

Wear natural fibers

Don't wear clothes made using synthetic fiber like nylon, polyester and acrylic. Budwig put great emphasis on the fact that her patients only wore natural fabrics such as cotton or satin, since they too can influence the magnetic field of our body.

Bed

Don't use on foam pillow and mattress. She recommended horsehair mattresses. Latex mattresses are the second choice. In any case, however, you should always replace mattresses that have metal spring cores.

CRT TV and mobile phones

These emit dangerous electromagnetic radiation, so do not use them. You can watch LCD and plasma TVs.

No left over

Food should be prepared fresh and eaten soon after preparation to maximize intake of health giving electrons and enzymes (Budwig, Cancer The Problem And The Solution).

Few Desserts recipes by Dr. Budwig

Fujiya delight

Ingredients for 3 people:
250 cc grape juice, 250 cc pure currant juice,
8g agar-agar, Quark-Flaxseed oil,
Milk, honey, vanilla cream

Preparation:

Heat the grape juice till it boils, then add the currant juice, agar-agar, stirring constantly for 5 minutes, and allow to cool. Now divide this mass to 3 narrow, tall cups, which have been rinsed with cold water. It is preferable if these cups have a bottom diameter of only 3- 4 cm. Refrigerate to cool. Now mix a Quark-Flaxseed oil cream with milk, honey and vanilla. Turn the red jelly upside down onto glass plates. The Quark-Flaxseed oil cream is placed on the top so that only the upper half is covered with the Quark-Flaxseed oil cream, so that top looks like the Snow caped Mount Fujiyama.

(The beautiful hotel with a gorgeous view of the Fujiyama is called "Fujiya", hence the dessert "Fujiya".)

(Oil-Protein Diet by Lothar Hirneise *available at http://www.hirneise.com/page-8/page-19/)*

Linovita-in-love in wine jelly

Ingredients: for 5 people:
250 cc of grape juice, 250 ccm of white wine,
8 agar-agar, 4 tablespoons of milk,
8 tablespoons of Flaxseed oil, 2 teaspoons of honey,
200-250 g of Quark, 2 liqueur glasses
Vodka, plum (Slibowitz) or cherry brandy or rum

Preparation:

The wine jelly is prepared by heating 250 cc of grape juice till it boils. Agar-agar is stirred with a little wine and placed in the boiling grape juice. Immediately remove from the cooking plate and add the remaining wine gradually with constant stirring. After about 5 minutes, the jelly mixture clears itself. You can now divide to approx. 5 glass bowls or champagne glasses. Immediately afterwards, mix the Quark-Flaxseed oil cream from Flaxseed oil, milk, honey and Quark. Finally, add 2 liqueur glasses of vodka or slibovitz or cherry brandy or rum into the Quark-Flaxseed oil cream. This Quark-Flaxseed oil mixture is evenly divided on the ready to-use bowls so that the Quark-Flaxseed oil cream partly sinks down in the middle. It is served after complete solidification.

(Oil-Protein Diet by Lothar Hirneise available at http://www.hirneise.com/page-8/page-19/)

Ice cream with cocoa

Ingredients:

3 tablespoons of Flaxseed oil, 3 tablespoons of milk,
1 tablespoon of honey, 100g of Quark, 100 g of hazelnuts,
2 tablespoons of cocoa

Preparation:

Quark, Flaxseed oil, milk and honey are mixed in the blender, then the hazelnuts are added, well blended and finally, cocoa is added to the mixture. Now pour the entire mixture into the ice-maker and place it in the fridge compartment of the refrigerator. This mixture with a nougat flavor gives the various combinations mentioned here the dark color contrast. For very ill people these preparations are very important, especially when there is a general lack of appetite.

(Oil-Protein Diet by Lothar Hirneise available at http://www.hirneise.com/page-8/page-19/)

ELDI oils

Dr. Budwig created unique ELDI oils, called electron differential oils after performing precise spectroscopic measurements of the light absorption in different oils - specifying that the oils contained pi-electron clouds from Flax oil, wheat germ oil plus vitamin-E in its natural complex, etheric oils and sulfhydryl groups.

Dr. Johanna Budwig said, "The sun is my preferred treatment modality, as is ELDI oil, used externally to stimulate the absorption of the long-wave band of the sun. I have used ELDI oils extensively since 1968 for body massage as well as in the selective application of oil packs. US pain institute has written somewhere: "What this crazy woman does with her ELDI oils, none of us manages to do via pain killers." Dr. Budwig has mentioned that if ELDI oil is not available, you may use Flax oil instead. *You can buy ELDI oils at: www.sensei.de*

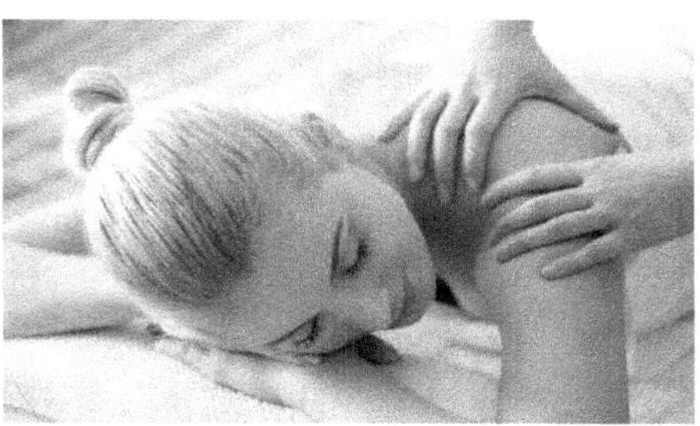

Massage Benefits

- Since ancient time massage has been part of cancer healing. Think of your lymphatics as a trash-disposal system for your body. Massage initiates lymphatic drainage, you push the trash out of your body and you're helping your immune system.
- Massage therapy is sometimes the first really pleasant touch a patient is able to experience.
- Massage also releases endorphins (our body's natural painkillers), stimulates lymph movement, and stretches tissues throughout the body. It's energizing, stimulating, and pretty good feeling.

ELDI oil plans:

A: For cancer patients in support of the energy level

    1. Full-body rubbings in the morning
    2. ELDI oil R enema with 200ml every 2-3 days
    3. Wrap at the "place of the happening"

B: For energetically weak patients

    1. Full-body rubbings in the morning and in the evening
    2. Enema: standard plan for ELDI oil R
    3. Wrap at the "place of the happening"
    4. Daily liver wrap with ELDI oil sage

Additional information:

- Make sure that you make once a week an (deep/high) enema with water or coffee.
- If you make daily coffee enemas, then start in the morning with the coffee enema and then with the ELDI R enema, but only if your energetic level allows you to make two enemas daily. Otherwise, only make the ELDI R enema. (Oil Protein Diet by Lothar Hirneise)

ELDI oils from SENSEI (www.sensei.de) are produced in a permanent cold chain in a European oil mill and marketed under the name of Electron Differentiation Oils. There are two qualities. A 6-star organic quality and a 5-star quality, which are produced exclusively for the IOPDF (www.iopdf.com).

Cost factor ELDI oils

Again and again we hear that for reasons of cost, patients use Flax seed oil instead of ELDI oil R for an enema. Please do not do so, because Flax seed oil does not react in the same way as ELDI oil R. Instead, use cheap ELDI oils from IOPDF or reduce the amount of oil.

Procedure –

Two times a day, i.e. morning and evening, rub ELDI Oil or Flax oil into the skin over the whole body, a bit more intensely on the shoulders, armpits and groin area (where plenty of lymphatic vessels are present) as well as the problem areas, such as the breast, stomach, liver, etc. Leave the oil on the skin for about 20 minutes and follow with a warm water shower without washing with soap. After 10 minutes take another shower, this time using a mild soap, and then relax for 15-20 minutes.

Once the body has been oiled and the ELDI Oil or Flax oil has penetrated the skin, the warm water will open the skin pores and the oil penetrates the skin more deeply. The second shower, where one washes with soap, cleanses the skin so that clothes and linen will not become overly soiled.

Oil Packs

Take a piece of cloth made of pure cotton. Cut to a size to fit the body part, such as the knee. Soak the cotton cloth with oil, place on the knee etc., cover it with a piece of polythene and wrap it up with an elastic bandage. Leave overnight. Remove in the morning and wash the knee; repeat in the evening. Keep applying the same procedure for weeks, you get good results. You also use Flax oil or castor oil for these local applications if you do not get ELDI oils . Dr Budwig generally recommended ELDI sage and should be used in the following indications:

- Tumors
- Painful skin areas
- Metastases
- Hepatic impairment and liver support
- Kidney problems
- Bladder disorders
- Intestinal cramps
- Lung disorders
- Bone disorders of all kinds

ELDI Oil Enema

Enemas are used in the Oil-Protein Diet exclusively for the energy intake and not for the purification of the intestine. Dr Budwig used to give ELDI oil or Flax oil enema to her serious patients. Budwig used to get immediate and miraculous results with the most seriously ill patients. Flax seed Oil enema also give similar results.

I recommend you to make the first enemas only with 100ml and then increase over several days to 250ml. Some patients have enemas with 500ml oil and positively reported on it. 500ml are however the absolute exception and mostly not necessary. Usually 250ml suffice.

Incidentally, smaller amounts are also easily introduced with an enema syringe instead of with an enema bucket. Enema syringes are available in sizes up to 350ml and are easy to handle.

Standard plan for ELDI oil R: Day 1 = 100ml, day 2 = 100ml, day 3 = 150ml, day 4 = 150ml, day 5 = 200ml, day 6 = 200ml and day 7 = 250ml.

From the seventh day, one remains at 250ml, and so long until the patient is significantly better. Then you can go back to 100ml - 150ml, always together with 1-2 daily whole body rubbings. (Oil Protein Diet by Lothar Hirneise)

Ingredients

- Enema pot
- Watch
- A bowl to collect oil when you are getting rid of bubbles.
- Towel and tissue
- RO filtered water
- ELDI oil or Flax oil
- Towel or Drip Stand

Procedure

Prepare a place near the toilet, so that if you can't hold the enema, you will be making a quick dash and the shorter distance is better.

Cleansing Enema with Plain water

First of all you should take a plain water enema. Purpose of this enema is cleaning of intestines. It is not a retention enema and is evacuated immediately. For this you may use 500-1000ml (2-4 cups) RO filtered water. As soon as the whole water is inside the rectum, go and sit on the commode and release the water slowly.

Take the oil enema immediately after the water enema

- Use advised (above) amount of ELDI or Flax oil. The oil should be at body temperature. The best test is to dip your little finger into the oil.
- Fill the oil into the enema pot. It takes at least 5 minutes for the bubbles to get out of the tube.
- The enema pot should be hanged on a drip stand about 2-3 feet above your body.
- You need to lubricate the nozzle and anus with Flax oil. When all is ready, lie on your right side in the fetal position. Insert the nozzle into the rectum slowly and carefully with your left hand, and un-pinch the tube.
- If you feel little uncomfortable when the oil is going in, pinch the tube, wait till the feeling passes away, then continue again.
- The oil is much more viscous and moves more slowly. You might need to hold the pot a bit higher to get it to run a bit quicker.
- Once the oil is in, wait and hold it for about 12 minutes. After that slowly turn yourself to left side and hold oil for another 12 minutes. You may listen to music while taking enema.
- When done, it is best to sit on the commode for about 15 minutes with something to read (Skelton).

Coffee Enema

Dr. Max Gerson introduced coffee enema back in the 1930s. In this enema about 500ml of coffee is pushed into rectum, this amount only reaches up to sigmoid colon. There is no loss of minerals and electrolytes in Coffee Enema because their absorption occurs well before sigmoid colon. Coffee enema is even safe for those who are allergic to coffee because it is not absorbed into the systemic circulation. You may take this enema once or twice. It has the following benefits:

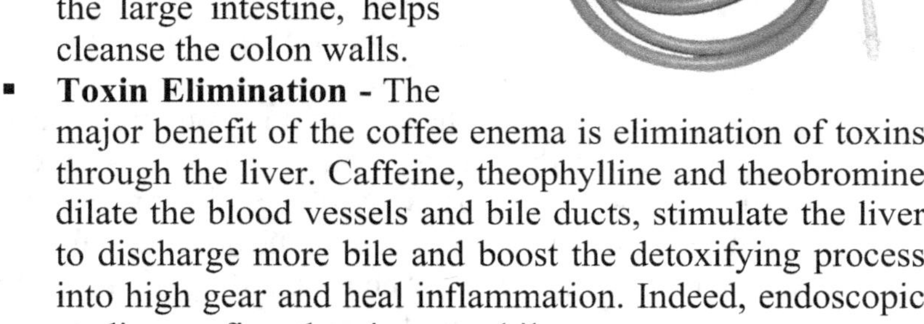

- **Powerful and Natural Pain Reliever**
- **Cleansing** - Coffee also acts as an astringent in the large intestine, helps cleanse the colon walls.
- **Toxin Elimination** - The major benefit of the coffee enema is elimination of toxins through the liver. Caffeine, theophylline and theobromine dilate the blood vessels and bile ducts, stimulate the liver to discharge more bile and boost the detoxifying process into high gear and heal inflammation. Indeed, endoscopic studies confirm they increase bile output.
- **Stimulates Liver -** Kahweol and cafestol palmitate found in coffee promote the activity of a key enzyme system called glutathione S-Transferase. This is an important mechanism in the detoxification of carcinogens, as the enzyme group is responsible for neutralizing free radicals. Coffee enema stimulates the activity of this system by 600- 700%.

Coffee Enema Procedure
- This enema is retained for 12-14 minutes, during this time blood circulates in liver three times and blood is purified. Coffee enema can be given several times a day, few patients take up to seven times a day. Normally if pain is not relieved it may be taken more than one time. You should relax while taking enema; you may listen to music or read newspaper while relaxing. The best time for coffee enema is either early morning after you passed motion or during the day time.

- Grind organic coffee beans. Put approx. 750ml of filtered water in a steal pan and bring it to boil. Add 2-5 heaped Tbsp coffee powder, 3 Tbsp is ideal. It is roughly 20-25grams. Let it continue to simmer for ten minutes or more and then turn off the burner. Allow it to cool down to a very comfortable, tepid temperature. Test it with your finger. It should be the same temperature as your body's temperature. Filter the coffee with fine mesh steal sieve into a jug. This is approximately 500ml.
- Pour 2 cups (500ml) of coffee into the enema pot. Be sure the plastic hose is clamped tightly. Now open the clamp and grasp, but do not close the clamp on the hose. Place the enema tip in the sink. Hold up the enema bag above the tip until the coffee begins to flow out. As soon as it starts flowing, quickly close the clamp. This expels any air in the tube.
- Lubricate the enema tip with a small amount of coconut oil or KY jelly. Create a comfortable and relaxing atmosphere. After a few days you will thoroughly enjoy this ritual.
- Light a candle, play some light music and most importantly, make sure you are comfortable and warm. We recommend placing a pillow with a washable cover under your head and lying down on a old towel.
- The position preferred is lying on your back. With the clamp closed hang the pot about 3 feet above your belly. We like to hang the enema pot on a drip stand.
- Insert the tip gently into anus and open the clamp slowly. You should relax and breathe. The coffee may take a few seconds to begin flowing. If you develop a cramp, close the hose clamp, turn from side to side and take a few deep breaths. The cramp will usually pass quickly. Usually nothing happens.
- When all the liquid is inside, close the clamp and remove it slowly. Retain the enema for 12- 14 minutes. You may remain lying on the floor.

- After 14 minutes or so, go to the toilet and empty your gut. Take your time. Wash the enema pot and tube thoroughly with soap and water.
- Take more potassium in the form of fruits and vegetable juices if you take coffee enema regularly (S.A.Wilsons.com).

Soda bicarb/ Epsom bath

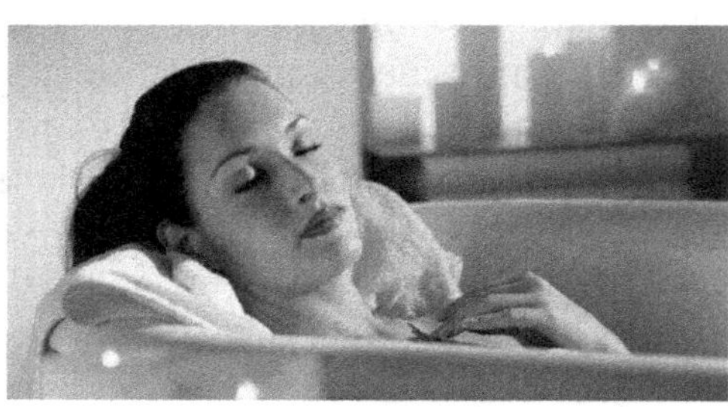

Detoxification of your body through bathing is an ancient remedy that anyone can perform in the comfort of your own home. Your skin is known as the third kidney, and toxins are excreted through sweating. Lothar Hirneise has given lot of importance to Soda bicarb bath. It is thought to assist you in eliminating toxins as well as making your body alkaline so your tumor cells may suffocate. Patient may take it once or even twice a day. Just add 2 cups of soda bicarb in your bath tub filled with warm water and relax in it for 30-40 minutes (Hirneise, 2005).

An Epsom salt bath is thought to assist your body in eliminating toxins as well as absorbing the magnesium and nutrients that are in the water. Soaking in Epsom salt actually helps replenish the body's magnesium levels, combating hypertension. The sulfate flushes toxins and helps form proteins in brain tissue and joints. Most of all, it will leave you relaxed, refreshed and awakened. Add Epsom salt two or three times a week or as advised.

Prepare your bath

- It is a 40 minutes ritual. The first 20 minutes are said to help your body remove the toxins, while the second 20 minutes are for absorbing the minerals from the water

- Fill your tub with comfortably hot water. Use a chlorine filter if possible.
- Add 2 cups or more of soda bicarb. It is known for its cleansing ability and even has anti-fungal properties. It also leaves skin very soft.
- Add 2-3 Tbsp ground ginger. While this step is optional, ginger can increase your heat levels, helping to sweat out more toxins. However, since it is heating the body, it may cause your skin to turn slightly red for a few minutes, so be careful with the amount you add. Depending on the capacity of your tub, anywhere from 1 Tbsp to 1/3 cup can be added (Herneise).
- Add aromatherapy oils. Again optional, but there are many oils that will make the bath an even more pleasant and relaxing experience (such as lavender), as well as those that will assist in the detoxification process (tea tree or eucalyptus oil). Around 20 drops is sufficient for a standard bath.
- For people weighing 50 Kg and up, add 2 cups or more Epsom Salt to a standard bath tub, two or three times a week.
- Swish all of the ingredients around in the tub, and then slip into the tub. You should start sweating within the first few minutes. If you feel too hot, start adding cold water into the tub until you cool off.
- Get out of the tub slowly and carefully. Your body has been working hard and you may get lightheaded or feel weak and drained. On top of that, the salts make your tub slippery, so stand with care.
- Drink plenty of water and relax in bed for a few minutes

Sun Therapy

Getting an adequate amount of sunshine is a critical part of Budwig protocol. Once the body has acquired the right oil-protein balance with the Cottage Cheeseand Flax oil, the body develops better capacity to absorb the healing photons from the sun. Remember that for healing of cancer high energy photons from the sun are very important. The sunshine is important to maintain adequate vitamin-D levels in our body. Vitamin-D is a powerful antioxidant that has been linked to preventing many diseases including cancer.

Dr. Budwig's focus was on the importance of photons from the sunbeams and their interaction with vital essential fats (linoleic and linolenic acid) in our body. It is the interaction of photons from the sun and the electrons in proper food that provide the synergistic effect on healing our body. Eating the electron rich Flax oil/Cottage Cheese mixture, must be connected with adequate exposure to sunlight.

There is nothing else on earth with a higher concentration of photons of the sun's energy than man. This concentration of the sun's energy is very much energetic point for humans, with their wave eminently suitable lengths - is improved when we eat electron rich essential oils, which in turn absorbs the photons in the form of electro-magnetic waves of sunbeams.

When you eat the FO/CC mixture, your body becomes a better antenna for the photons from the sunbeam. Your body develops a better ability to absorb the energy from the sun and Transfer it to your cells to perform their vital functions. You become energized at a deep level, and when this happens cancer is healed itself.

It is red light that penetrates deeper in the tissues. In 1968 Dr. Budwig used 695 nm ruby (red) laser light with success to radiate healthy surrounding cancer tissues in cancer patients.

Rebounder

Your body has about 60 trillion cells. The gravitational pull involved in bouncing on a "Rebounder" squeezes out toxins. Then, during the brief weightless period when the body is suspended in the air, the lower pressure in the cell promotes the movement of nutrients into the cells. Bouncing also has a pumping action of lymphatic system. Thus the flow of materials to and from cells is improved. It is like getting every cell in your body to exercise.

Oil-Protein Diet while travelling

- In her Oil-Protein Diet Cookbook, Dr. Budwig writes: "While traveling, you can always care for yourself with Linomel and hot or cold milk, and/or fruit juices."
- If you are eating a salad in a restaurant, never take the finished dressings, but use olive oil and vinegar. The chance not to take Trans fats is at the least.
- If you want something to be fried, ask the cook to put it in coconut fat or butter. Butter is present in every kitchen.
- Budwig also recommends eating various types of fresh fish to replace the Flax oil and Quark when travelling. You can protect yourself against harm while travelling by ordering fresh fish such as trout, pike, carp and other fresh fish. However, canned (tinned) fish, also shrimps, prawn and other items which frequently contain artificial coloring agents and harmful chemical preservatives, must be strictly avoided.
- Do not eat the "muesli" in hotels. They are mostly denatured carbohydrates.
- Do not use polyunsaturated oils (Flax seed oil, Oil, pumpkin seed oil, etc.) which are kept at room temperature and all contain Tran's fatty acids.

For a long vacation

During your long stay travelling away from home, it is really simple to keep up with the Budwig diet, all that is needed was a little bit of preplanning. You may have a fridge and electric tea kettle in the hotel room, or you carry a ice chest.

Wash all fruits and veggies and make enough juice for the travel day and one more day. You should carry a bowl, fork, spoon, sharp knife, and hand blender, nuts, oatmeal and tea. You carry Flax oil, cottage cheese, fruits and veggies in a ice chests for travel.

If you have "eaten something", especially too many carbohydrates in the form of potatoes, rice, noodles or even a "not so healthy dessert/cake", then you should take a walk immediately after eating. (Healing Cancer Naturally)

Making Quark

Quark is a very popular and delicious cheese in Germany. You may find many recipes of making Quark on Google. I am giving you a simple recipe here. In this recipe you will learn how it is easy to make your own homemade Quark.

Ingredients

- 1 liter milk preferably <2% fat
- 500ml cultured buttermilk
- Cheese cloth

Instructions

- In a large glass bowl add milk and buttermilk. Stir well and cover with a clean kitchen towel.
- Let this sit at room temperature for 24 hours. The mixture will thicken slightly.
- Heat the oven to 125^0 F and shut off. Set the bowl uncovered into the oven for about 45 min. The mixture will change to yogurt like texture.
- Add a Cheese cloth to a colander and set on a large bowl.

- Pour the milk mixture into the colander, twist the ends and let drain for about 1 ½ to 2 hours.
- The Quark will be in the towel and the whey will be in the bowl. One liter milk usually yields 200gms of Quark.

Making Cottage Cheese

In some places good quality Cottage Cheese is also not available and you need to make your own. Today I am giving you a very good recipe for home made cottage cheese.

Ingredients

- 1 liter natural, low-fat cow's milk preferably <2% fat
- 1/3 cup Vinegar
- Cold water

Instructions

- Mix 1/3 cup of vinegar in 2 cups of water and keep aside. Diluted vinegar yields soft cheese. You may also use diluted lemon juice.
- Boil the milk in a heavy bottomed pan over medium heat, stirring frequently making sure milk does not burn on the bottom of the pan. As the milk comes to a boil, remove the pan from the gas burner and place it on kitchen counter.
- Now add about a glass of cold water to bring the milk's temperature down to about 75-80 degrees Celsius. We want to curdle the milk at this temperature, so we get a soft cheese.
- Then add little (about 1-2 Tbsp) diluted vinegar slowly and stir the milk gently. After 10 seconds, add little vinegar slowly and stir the milk. Go on adding vinegar until the curd will start separating from the whey. Remember you should curdle the milk slowly.
- Once the cheese has completely separated from the whey, add a glass of cold water and drain the whey using a stainless steel strainer.

- Now Transfer the curdled cheese into a suitable container and blend thoroughly with electric hand blender until you get very smooth and thick creamy cheese. If the cheese is dry, add a little milk while blending. This is your home made cottage cheese.

Buckwheat

Dr. Budwig highly recommended buckwheat in her healing diet. Contrary to its name, this seed is not related to wheat. Buckwheat is a gluten free power food!

Buckwheat is supercharged with health-boosting nutrients and phytochemicals, including B-vitamins, magnesium, manganese, phosphorus, zinc, copper, potassium, and selenium. It is also one of the best natural sources of rutin and D-chiro-Inositol, two phytochemicals that have been associated with a number of interesting health benefits. It is the best source of high-quality, easily digestible proteins. This makes it an excellent meat substitute. What's more, buckwheat grouts (the hulled kernels) are generally well tolerated and rarely cause allergic reactions or other adverse effects in humans. These gluten-free kernels can be served as an alternative to rice or made into delicious buckwheat porridge.

Studies have shown that populations eating diets high in fiber-rich whole grains and seeds, like buckwheat, consistently have lower risk for colon cancer. Research reported at the American Institute for Cancer Research (AICR) International Conference on Food, Nutrition and Cancer, by Rui Hai Liu, M.D., Ph.D., and his colleagues at Cornell University shows that buckwheat, contain many powerful phytonutrients that can fight cancer.

Energy Healing

Mild exercise

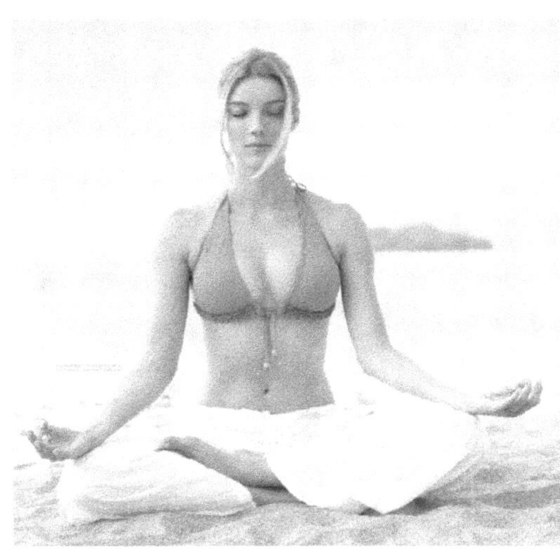

Patient can do mild exercise and remain active if his condition permits. He can go for a walk or do light yoga in the open terrace or garden under the healing and refreshing sunshine. Patient can jog for a few minutes after lunch or dinner. It is very beneficial for cancer patient. But if patient is serious and has metastasis, he should not jog, better he should relax in his house.

Patient can keep himself busy in many activities like sitting in garden enjoying nature, visualization, listening music, reading, laughing, chatting with friends etc. Stress, depression, anxiety, anger and fear can be very damaging to him. Share your feelings with your life partner or a best friend.

You should try your best to remove stress and negative thoughts and balance the flow of energy "prana" or "chi" in your body. Do meditation, Emotional Freedom Technique EFT, Qigong, Reiki, Acupuncture, Acupressure, Sun Salutation etc. to heal your body, mind and spirit.

Meditation

Meditation is a means of Transforming the mind. Meditation practices are techniques that encourage and develop concentration, clarity, positivity, and relaxation of the body and mind. Do any simple meditation for relaxation. Meditation stimulates pineal gland (*piyush granthi*) to shower melatonin hormone. Melatonin controls circadian rhythm and induces restorative sleep. Its powerful antioxidant effect offers important enhancements to the brain and nervous system, helping protect against age-related damage. Melatonin is power anti-stress and anticancer hormone.

Yoga Nidra

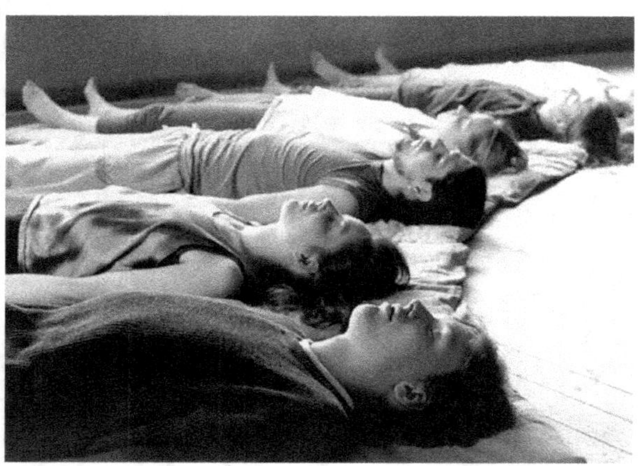

It is divine sleep with alertness. In 15 minute yoga nidra session, you relax in a fully supported shavasan, limbs limp, breath quiet, thoughts drifting by. In the distance, the teacher's voice blends with the sound of Tibetan bells. All traces of the day fade away, time stops, and stillness washes over the body. Yoga nidra is a systematic method of complete relaxation, holistically addressing our physiological, neurological, and subconscious needs.

How long should you take this protocol?

If all is well patient feels better and tumor start to shrink within a 3 or 4 months, if he follows treatment religiously and honestly. He may be cured in one or two years. **It is recommended that the Budwig protocol and full diet is followed for at least five years.** Even after that he should maintain healthy eating and life style.

Dr. Budwig has clearly mentioned that if you do not get the desired success, do not blame the protocol, rather try to find out your mistakes and correct them. The threshold between winning and losing is very small, and even a minor mistake can unbalance the complete healing process.

Juicing for the Budwig Protocol

"Juicing", making your own fresh juices, is one of the important cornerstones of the Budwig Protocol. There is no point in overloading on one fruit or vegetable juice; so try to get plenty of variety in the juices you drink.

Juices specifically recommended by Budwig include carrot, celery and apple, beet and apple, radish, cherry, grape, pomegranate and red currant and stinging nettle.

Mix and combine your juices to taste. Juices are best made with good, fresh and preferably organic fruit and vegetables. They should be drunk as fresh as possible to ensure the vitamins and enzymes are still active. It is always best to press it yourself for that meal.

Nettle juice is rich in vitamin C and always been a folk remedy for cleansing the blood. Almost all fruit and vegetables, leaves such as spinach, chard or watercress or even wheat and barley grass can be pressed.

Budwig Diet Juicing Routine

- Early morning you must have a glass of **sauerkraut juice**.
- **Breakfast:** Juice can be used to moisten ground linseed or add flavor to the Quark-Flax seed oil cream for breakfast in muesli or add a cup of juice to the ground Flax seed, Quark-Flax seed oil cream, liquidize the fresh fruits and berries and use a cup of juice to make a smoothie.
- **10 A.M.** Take a glass of vegetable juice.
- **Lunch** Juice can be used to add variety to the Quark-linseed oil cream in desserts

- **3 P.M.** Possibly grape, cherry, pomegranate juice, orange juice.
- **3:30 P.M.** Pineapple or papaya juice.

Juicing Tips

- The cruciferous family, cabbages, kohlrabi, turnips, kale, broccoli and watercress all taste good pressed with apple and if you add some sort of sharp whole citrus fruits such as orange, the juiced peel increases the antioxidants and tang.
- Tomatoes, peppers, celery and cucumber are great with apple and beetroot, try a little garlic and/or onion or even chili peppers.
- Apples, pears, rose-hips or berries are great.
- Carrots and beetroot are great for color and flavor.
- Ginger and lemon are the very best for giving juice a real lift and loads of extra goodness. In a vegetable juice, chilies are surprisingly good.
- Lemon pressed with apple and pear helps keep the juice form going brown.
- Wheat or barley grass grown to about 7 inches or 200 mm high are amazing sources of nutrients and ideal for an extra shot of greens in your juice. Wheat is perhaps richer in nutrients; barley tastes nicer.
- Spinach and Swiss Chard make sweeter, less pungent green juices than you might expect.

Juicers

You will need a juicing machine. Whichever juicer you choose, you will be amazed at how good your own home-made fresh juice is. Within reason the more money you spend on a juicer, the better the juice, pressed at cooler temperatures and the more juice is extracted from the pulp – which makes it more cost-effective. Some machines are much easier to clean than others. Budwig prefers masticating juicer. Kuvings B1700 and Omega J8006 are the best, economic and masticating juicers available.

Juicing on the Budwig Diet is going to be a big part of your life so get a good one (Skelton).

How do I recognize a good Flax seed oil?

Good Flax seed oil is unfortunately dependent on many factors. The IOPDF assigns a star for each fulfilled criterion. The best oil has thus 6 stars and the worst gets no star. Let us look at the 6 criteria in detail:

Criterion 1: Cooling chain

Studies have shown that, in addition to processing the Flax seed, cooling is the most important criterion for a good Flax seed oil. So buy only Flax seed oil stored in a refrigerated rack and kept in a permanent cold chain. If you shop through the Internet, the Flax seed oil must be delivered in a Styrofoam packaging and as fast as possible.

Criterion 2: Local Flax seed

Weekly shipping on ships and sometimes additional chemicals used can cause great damage to Flax seed. Therefore, make sure that you only buy Flax seed oil whose Flax seed comes from the country where you are living or at least from the same continent. This normally can be seen at the seal.

Criterion 3: Omega-3 fatty acid content

The Oil-Protein Diet is about linolenic acid (omega-3). Buy Flax seed oil with a high amount of linolenic acid. Depending in which country you are living the range can be between 55% - 63%.

Criterion 4: Organic quality

It makes a big difference whether Flax seed grows in biologically controlled soil or in soils of conventional agriculture. So buy only Flax seed oils with organic quality, unless you know the oil mill personally and know what Flax seed the mill is processing.

Criterion 5: glass bottle

Flax seed oil and electron differentiation oils are available in glass and plastic bottles or in canisters, which are mostly made of tinplate. Consumers should only buy oils in glass bottles. Avoid plastic bottles, as they may contain highly toxic softeners.

Criterion 6: Light

Flax seed oil should be packaged and stored in a light-proof package. Therefore, only buy bottles in dark brown or dark green bottles. (Oil Protein Diet by Lothar Hieneise)

Linomel

Linomel is an invention by Dr Budwig. Freshly crushed Flax seed is mixed with honey and milk powder so that the crushed Flax seed is more stable. There is no doubt that freshly crushed Flax seed is more valuable, but also has the disadvantage that you do it yourself and clean the grinder afterwards. That is why Linomel still has an existence right. Do not buy crushed Flax seed in the shop as the chance that these contain Tran's fatty acids is 100%.

Is there an alternative to Linomel?

- Freshly crushed Flax seed is an alternative. This must be eaten immediately after the meal, otherwise it will oxidize.
- Make your own Linomel. Mix 6 tablespoons freshly crushed Flax seed with a tablespoon of honey. Small tip: Grind the Flax seed, e.g. in a coffee grinder, and set the grinder to coarse. So it mixes better with the honey.

(Oil Protein Diet by Lothar Hieneise)

Questions and Answers

How do I store Flax seed oil?

Generally cool. Best at 5^0-10^0 (Fahrenheit 41-50) in the refrigerator. Always keep the Flax seed oil bottles upright and never lay them down as they may cause faster oxidation.

Should I now buy low fat Quark or Quark with 20% or 40% fat?

Only a Quark with as little fat (less than 2%) is optimal. Quark is about sulfur-containing amino acids. Less fat means more amino acids.

Can Quark be replaced with tofu, yoghurt or soya?

Absolutely no.

Is there an alternative to Quark?

In many books or on the Internet, it is always claimed that there are alternatives to Quark, such as e.g., yogurt, soy or whey protein (which you should never use!). This is wrong. There is absolutely no good substitute for Quark. The only alternative (although it has a slightly different composition like Quark) is Cottage Cheese with as little fat as possible. This should only be used if no Quark is available.

Can I eat cheese?

Basically yes, but in moderation and with the exception of cream cheese and fresh cheese. Only raw milk/hard cheese is permitted. Cheese of sheep or goat is preferable.

Can I eat raisins and dates?

Yes, raisins and dates are allowed in small quantities.

Which fat can be used for frying?

Only coconut fat.

Can I use olive oil?

Theoretically, you can use any organic oils with salad. Dr Budwig preferred Flax seed oil, pumpkin seed oil, wheat germ oil, poppy oil, and thistle oil are also permitted, but do not heat. Oleolox may be heated for two minutes.

Can I drink coffee?

No.

Can soya and oatmeal be eaten?

Dr Budwig wrote several times that oat flakes, soy flakes, yeast flakes and other flakes are permitted. But today I just say that you buy only high quality organic "flakes".

Can I eat bread?

Dr Budwig has recommended her patients to eat no bread during acute tumor phases. Instead, she recommended full-grain rice waffles or Ezekiel bread as an alternative.

Can cows or soy milk be drunk?

No, drinking any milk is forbidden in the Oil-Protein Diet.

Can noodles be eaten?

In the literature of Dr Budwig nearly always did not allow cancer patients to eat noodles. The reason is that noodles are made of flour, eggs and oil. Flour has the disadvantage that it is basically a fast-digesting sugar and mostly the producers use cheap oils. Energetically speaking, noodles are "not really full with electrons". Unfortunately, you are worsening the already bad adrenaline - insulin ratio of a cancer patient.

Which milk can be used for the Quark?

Dr Budwig recommended raw milk. Unfortunately these are nowadays difficult to buy anywhere. Alternatively, pasteurized milk is also okay. All other varieties of milk, such as ultra-heat-treated or homogenized (long life or full cream), are prohibited.

Budwig- Compatible Pain Therapies

Items written in **CAPITALS** are more significant. Foods for managing & healing cancer pain

Flax seed oil mixed with Quark (Oil Protein Muesli)

Eldi oils (developed by Dr. Johanna Budwig)

A glass of organic **sparkling wine or champagne** with linomel.

KOMBUCHA is a lightly effervescent fermented drink of sweetened black tea that is used as a functional food. It is produced by fermenting the tea using a symbiotic colony of bacteria and yeast, or "SCOBY". Kombucha contains over 50 different kinds of probiotics, enzymes, amino acids and vitamins. Kombucha is typically produced by placing a culture in a sweetened tea, as sugar is necessary for fermentation. A kombucha scoby (also known as a starter culture, mother etc.) is a necessary component if you wish to make kombucha from tea (Schmid, Healing Cancer Naturally).

Cherries

Cherries can help adults maintain an active lifestyle by relieving pain and inflammation. By averting cancer and protecting the nervous system, a diet containing tart cherries may help ensure a future, free from debilitating illness. Both sweet and tart cherries are a good source of fiber, vitamin C and potassium. Tart cherries, but not sweet cherries or tart cherry juice, are also an excellent source of vitamin A. Cherries contain a variety of phytochemicals contributing both color and antioxidant activity.

The fruit's dark red color comes from their high content of anthocyanins, which are antioxidants. Strong evidence from several studies has revealed that cherry's anthocyanins offer powerful relief against inflammation and pain (Schmid, Healing Cancer Naturally).

Hydroxycinnamic acid and perillyl alcohol, a phytochemical from the monoterpene family, provide great antioxidant power to cherries. Benefits are as follows:

Preventing and Fighting Cancer

In addition to providing welcome relief from inflammation, antioxidant-rich tart cherries also hold a lot of promise in protecting against cancer.

Supporting Melatonin Levels and Brain Health

Tart cherries are one of the few food sources of melatonin, a chemical released in the body by the pineal gland that is intimately connected with circadian rhythms, or the regulation of the sleep-wake cycle. Melatonin also acts as a powerful antioxidant, providing neuroprotective and immune-modulating effects.

Tempeh & FERMENTED SOY products - reduces inflammation

Apple cider vinegar & honey

- One 8 oz glass of cool water
- One cup full of apple cider vinegar
- One Tbsp of organic honey
- Stir well and sip slowly.

Nutritional yeast flakes (Nerve Food): pain stemming from neuritis (inflammation of a nerve) may respond quickly to nutritional yeast, a rich source of B vitamins

Herbs & supplements (organic or wild-crafted)

- ESSIAC
- ALOE VERA
- Maria Treben's herbs
- NONI JUICE
- Mushrooms: MAITAKE (effective in 83% of patients), CORDYCEPS, shiitake & reishi
- DL-PHENYLALANINE (an amino acid)

- Tian Xian paste
- PURPLE CONE FLOWER
- LOBELIA
- Angelica
- Pau d'Arco Tea
- Goldenseal root poultices
- Echinacea (anti-bacterial, anti-viral, anti-parasitic and stimulate lymph flow)
- Mistletoe
- Chaparral
- Turmeric/Curcumin, burdock, ginger - Pain caused by inflammation
- Boswellia Serrata, white willow bark, ginger, green-lipped mussel extract: these anti-inflammatory herbs work against pain triggered by inflammation, inhibit pro-inflammatory mediators, particularly leukotrienes.
- Bromelain/Pineapple
- Oregano Oil (oregano oil can have the same effect on the body as morphine)
- SINUSBUSTER (a nasal spray)
- Hot chili pepper powder in water
- AMYGDALIN/LAETRILE/Vitamin B17

Mind-body approaches to healing cancer pain
- EFT (Emotional Freedom Technique)
- VISUALIZATION, MEDITATION, YOG NIDRA & RELAXATION TECHNIQUES
- Laughter
- Prayer
- Tai chi or chi kung (aka taiji or qigong) - not only relieve the pain but lower the fever within fifteen to thirty minutes, sometimes up to two degrees.
- Foot / hand reflexology and massage
- Acupuncture and Reiki
- Bioptron light therapy
- Kinesiology
- Biotape

- TENS (Transcutaneous Electrical Nerve Stimulation) Therapy

Detoxification approaches to managing cancer pain

- Alkalizing one's body via fresh juicing and alkaline foods.
- Sodium bicarbonate is also strongly alkalizing.
- Coffee enemas and other detox methods
- Dental detox
- Castor oil packs
- Hot baths with Epsom salts
- Water drinking
- Charcoal

Misc.

- Honey packs
- Homeopathic remedies-- particularly Aconitum (1M or 10M dose)
- Exercise
- MSM

Sodium bicarbonate as pain reliever

Sodium bicarbonate is an easily available alkalizer and has been used for many applications, including cancer treatment. Sodium Bicarbonate has attractive and potent analgesic qualities. Dr. Tullio Simoncini recommends that his cancer patients, undergoing his bicarbonate protocols usually via IV administration, take 1 Tsp. of sodium bicarbonate mixed in water per day, for pain control as well as to assist in keeping an alkaline internal environment (Schmid, Healing Cancer Naturally).

Remedy for Bone pain

Bitter apricot kernels may help in the bone pains. Apricots contain vitamin B-17. Make sure you are getting papaya or pineapple every day. Grind the apricot seeds in the coffee grinder with the pumpkin seeds. You need one seed for every 5 kilos of body weight (Schmid, Healing Cancer Naturally). Also take a

Tsp pumpkin seeds as a natural source of zinc. Zinc is Transport vehicle for vitamin B-17.

Budwig's advice for very ill cancer patients

Simple measures to help the very weak and/or unable to eat cancer patients at a very late stage of their disease frequently are unable to eat much. For this type of person, Dr Johanna Budwig told to focus on these treatment approaches:

- **Total body massage** with Flax seed or Eldi oils and Flax seed or Eldi oils enemas;
- **Freshly pressed juices** only and if possible feed the FOCC in various variations spread over the course of the day.
- **Sun Therapy** as much as possible.
- **Champagne - an elixir for ill** - Dr Budwig used to prescribe alcohol for patients, whose energy level was very low (a maximum of 1-2 glasses a day) Both champagne and wine exert a positive influence on the intestinal environment. Ethanol rapidly supplies energy to the body but unlike glucose can't be utilized by cancer cells. Ethanol thus is an optimal energy source which doesn't feed the tumor for debilitated cancer patients. Ethanol also stimulates the appetite which typically will be near-absent in patients at this stage.

  Stay outside in the open as much as possible by combining it with barefoot (or any bare skin) contact with the earth or grass (Schmid, healingcancernaturally.com).

Nausea and vomiting due to Cancer

- **Herbs - Black Horehound** (Ballota nigra) and **German Chamomile** (Matricaria recutita) are particularly helpful. Both are relaxants to the intestinal area. German Chamomile has relaxing, anti-inflammatory, anti-nausea, and pain relief actions. **Ginger** is widely used to relieve severe nausea and prevent colds. Ginger also aids in metabolism."

- **Acupressure** - The easiest acupressure point to find for treating nausea is on the back of the mandible/jaw; just below the ear - the vertical part - push forward... as if you're pushing the lower jaw out like an under bite.

- **Acupuncture**

- **EFT**

- **Homeopathy** - In a much diluted dose, Ipeca becomes a remedy to control nausea and vomiting.

- **Qigong**
- **Guided imagery**
- **Music**
- **Hypnosis, hypnotherapy and biofeedback**
- **Color therapy**

(Schmid, Healing Cancer Naturally)

Painful adhesions after abdominal surgery

- **MSM (Methyl sulfonyl methane)** - MSM softens and can even dissolve scar tissue and frequently works as a powerful pain reliever, including with adhesions.
- **Castor oil packs** - have dissolved abdominal scar tissue from adhesions after applying them for an hour each day for about two months.
- **Foot reflexology** - Erika Herbst's landmark book "Die Heilkunst von Morgen" (The Healing Arts of Tomorrow) reports on one Wilhelm Heuser who after five abdominal surgeries had considerable discomfort and pain from adhesions. Since his doctors couldn't help, he tried foot reflexology with which he had had excellent results for other complaints. With adhesions the (external and internal) scars must be well supplied with blood so that the tissues stay or re-become elastic. For four months he had daily foot reflexology sessions (possibly self-applied) and now is free of complaints from adhesions and always

feeling well. He also changed to a whole foods diet and took bee pollen and Silica on a daily basis. This lifestyle very considerably improved his general health.

- **Kelley Eidem's recipe** Author Kelley Eidem suggests using his habanero peppers/garlic recipe together with one or two Zymessence (found online and perhaps at health food stores) three times a day taken with 8 ounces of water on an empty stomach plus some digestive enzymes with food.

- In cases of intractable pain, EFT (Emotional Freedom Technique) has often provided extremely effective pain relief (Healingcancernaturally.com).

Lymphedema Treatment

- Lymphedema is difficult to treat. Conservative treatments such as bandaging, proper skin care, compression garments, and exercises are some general methods of care. There is no easy surgical treatment for lymphedema. Surgical procedures have been tried in general, few of them work well in the long term; some make the condition even worse, and more difficult to treat.

- **Detoxification** Detoxify as much as possible. Use detoxifying baths such as Epsom salt baths.

- **EMF avoidance**

- **Increase circulation** - use of rebounder, massage (manual lymph drainage) and elevation can also be helpful. Take the enzyme preparation Wobenzym as directed on the label.

- Diet, foods or food components - Budwig's Healing Diet

- **Nutritional support** such as **bromelain** found in raw pineapples, and **oligomeric proanthocyanidins (OPCs)** found in grape seed and other sources. Bromelain is said to reduce swelling & break up immune complexes that cause inflammation.

- **Green power foods and drinks** such as daily freshly pressed organic wheatgrass, celery and parsley juice and spirulina reportedly helped a woman cure her lymphedema.
- **Herbs** - Butcher's broom, ginger tea, sweet clover (*Melilotus*) ointment contains coumarin which stimulates lymph flow & speeds skin wound healing. Butcher's broom alternated with horse chestnut works well. **Red clover** (which also has anti-cancer properties) as well as fenugreek appear to be helpful as well.
- **Cabbage leaf packs**
- **Energy medicine & energetic approaches**
- Homeopathy (such as the remedy called Serum Anguillae), EFT, chi kung (both of which can be self-applied), acupuncture and similar "energetic" approaches to healing aim at increasing the flow of life force energy and/or overcoming energetic blockages.
- **Healing stones**
- **Visualization** -Visualize a healthy arm/leg and/or the lymph nodes
- **Red Light treatment**

(Schmid, Healing Cancer Naturally)

Natural Cough Remedies

Reducing exposure to irritants is an important means to avoid arousing the cough reflex. Adequate hydration is essential to avoid drying of the membranes. **Simple steam inhalation** can be adequate for reducing coughs due to irritation of the respiratory airway below the throat.

Cough Suppressants

Coughs originating above the voice box can be appropriately treated with soothing demulcents. Licorice (Glycyrrhiza) extract is usually thought of as simply a demulcent with a pleasant flavor, but its derivatives have been shown to have a central antitussive effect similar to codeine. Licorice is also considered to be a sedative expectorant. In addition its constituents have shown antiviral and immune-stimulating effects. About 30 drops of the fluid extract is used per dose. (Every 15 drops of any fluid extract is equivalent to 1 gram of the powdered herbal remedy.) However, long-term use of large amounts of licorice is hazardous since this can lead to potassium loss and high blood pressure.

An antitussive that works by reducing irritation of the respiratory membrane at or below the voice box is wild cherry bark (Prunus). Wild cherry bark is effective for nervous coughs and is often used in short-term infectious cases or when convalescing. The compound prunasin in wild cherry bark can be toxic in large amounts but in smaller quantities relieves the irritation of the mucosa and thereby alleviates coughing. From 20-40 drops of the fluid extract is normally taken. About 1.3 ounce of good quality bark must be used and extracted by 1 quart of room temperature water (not by boiling) to make the tea which is taken in 2 ounce doses.

Marshmallow root For anyone suffering from a sore throat, cough or cold, marshmallow root can be taken orally to reduce pain, swelling and congestion. Its antitussive properties and mucilage abilities allow it to decrease irritation of the throat, reduce swelling in the lymph nodes, speed up healing time and reduce aggravating dry coughing. This is exactly the reason that marshmallow extract is added to many cough syrups and throat lozenges — it's one of the most effective natural cough remedies.

It also seems to help stop the urge to cough and facilitates with the process of producing more saliva, allowing it help reduce symptoms of dry mouth. It can safely be used by people with chronically low levels of salivary flow and chronic coughs.

Marshmallow is especially effective at beating a cold or the flu when combined with other anti-inflammatory and antibacterial herbs and essential oils for sore throat, such as slippery elm and echinacea or lemon, myrrh, oregano, cypress, and frankincense essential oils. When combined, these target the underlying cause of the sickness (including bacteria) and coat the throat to ease discomfort.

Demulcents and Expectorants

Demulcents contain mucilaginous components that are used for their soothing effect on irritations of the membrane lining the throat. Coltsfoot leaf (Tussilago), Marshmallow root (Althea) and slippery elm bark (Ulmus) are sources of mucilage for allaying inflammation and alleviating coughs. Water extracts of Mullein flowers (Verbascum), besides providing demulcent and expectorant effects, inhibit influenza viruses. Mullein leaf extract is also used for its demulcent mucilage in irritation from persistent coughs, whether dry or productive.

Flax seed tea is another effective remedy to cure common cold and cough. You can boil flaxseeds until it thickens and strain it. Add a few drops of lime juice and honey to it and consume the mixture for cold and cough relief.

Sedative Expectorants

Sedative expectorants are used when the membrane is dry, sensitive, reddened, and swollen or when there is thick, scanty, adherent mucus in the airway tubes. These remedies have an antitussive action by increasing the amount of respiratory fluid, thereby producing a soothing effect on the bronchial membranes, and by decreasing the thickness of membrane secretions, thus facilitating their removal.

Ipecac is used both to liquefy thick, tenacious mucus from the airways and to relieve spasms of the respiratory tubes, particularly spasms from croup. It reduces bronchial swelling and distress, and the coughing becomes easier. The main application for ipecac is in bronchial congestion with a dry, irritable cough. Ipecac is especially indicated when there is irritation with a continued effort to clear the larynx. It may be the best expectorant for acute conditions when taken in small, frequent doses insufficient to cause nausea. An appropriate dose for the syrup of ipecac used as an expectorant would be 4-8 drops given every two hours. This is much less than the single 1-2 tablespoon dose taken as an emetic.

Bloodroot is used for harsh, dry coughs with constriction or constant irritation or tickling in the throat. Its alkaloids produce a direct antitussive effect on the CNS cough center. Bloodroot is stimulant to the bronchial membranes, overcoming congestion and increasing membrane secretions. Considered too harsh a remedy for young children, it is used for acute or chronic bronchitis or laryngitis (inflammation of the voice box) when membranes are atonic after active inflammation has subsided. The expectorant dose of the tincture is 5-30 drops, while 1-3 teaspoons will cause vomiting.

Lobelia is used in cases of respiratory spasm such as croup, as well as coughs due to irritation. It is specific for bronchial asthma. It promotes expectoration and improves respiration in acute bronchitis with coughing, especially where there is thick mucus with tightness and difficulty breathing. The potent antispasmodic action of lobelia helps avoid trapping of the sputum and assists in its expulsion. The expectorant dose of the tincture is from 5-20 drops, whereas the dose causing vomiting is from 1/2-2 teaspoons. Lobelia is often combined with cayenne when used as an antispasmodic.

Bronchial Relaxants

Respiratory tract irritation that causes coughing also causes the bronchi to narrow. Some sedative expectorants used for dry, spasmodic coughs help reduce the tightness while not producing gastric irritation. **Pleurisy root** (Asclepias) is used for acute bronchitis or influenza with a tight, painful cough and difficult respiration. When there is a general reduction in respiratory secretions and the chest is sore from coughing, it is most beneficial, especially in children. Taken hot, it acts as a diaphoretic to help control fevers where there is hot, dry skin. One ounce of the powdered root is extracted with one quart of hot water and a tea cupful is taken every 2-3 hours. In pleurisy the cough is short, due to the pain, and hacking. This type of cough provides no benefit and should be ameliorated with an appropriate combination containing pleurisy root.

Sundew (Drosera) is called for in similar acute or chronic cases where the cough is dry, irritable, and persistent, particularly if it is hoarse, resonant, or explosive. Nervous coughs or spasmodic coughs such as during measles or after whooping cough are treated with small doses to advantage. The dose of the fluidextract is from 5-20 drops. Sundew and pleurisy root are also useful for the persistent cough following influenza.

Lungwort (Sticta) is used in dry, persistent, irrigative coughs with rasping and wheezing. Where there is asthmatic tightness or spasms such as in croup, it is useful. The exhaustive cough of acute bronchitis or laryngitis with short, sharp hacking and darting pains or muscular soreness in the chest indicates its usefulness. Pain in the back of the neck and shoulders or shoulder blades from coughing is another indication for lungwort. **Red clover** flowers (Trifolium) are used for dry, irritable coughs due to irritation of the larynx or bronchi and for spasmodic coughs such as occur with measles.

Where coughing is associated with asthma or emphysema, more potent remedies for opening the air tubes in the lungs should be used along with expectorants to provide relief for either dry or productive coughs.

Ephedra (Ephedra) is a potent antispasmodic like lobelia which, unlike lobelia, is not an expectorant. However, ephedra is useful for coughs associated with airway spasms. In these cases it is always combined with other remedies. Unfortunately, ephedra is likely to cause rapid heart rate and raise the blood pressure (Francis Brinker ND, Healthy.net).

Budwig Diet & Protocol - In Brief

This is raw organic diet with lot of Flax oil and Juices. Consume only clean or RO filtered water. To get the best results, proper guidance is strongly recommended. Below are brief guidelines of the Budwig Diet you don't have to consume all the foods on this list. This information is from Dr. Budwig's books.

First thing in the morning – One glass of sauerkraut juice, preferably raw & homemade. Raw unheated kraut has enzymes, probiotics and vitamins which help the digestive system, metabolize foods & improve immunity.

Just before breakfast - green or herbal tea

Breakfast – First blend 3 Tbsp. Flax oil, 3 Tbsp. milk and a Tsp real honey; then gradually add 6 Tbsp. Quark or Cottage Cheese and blend. Garnish in layers. Add 2 Tbsp freshly ground Flax seeds n a bowl, then add a layer of crushed fresh fruits, then pour oil cheese mixture and put raw nuts on top. Afterward, if hungry, choose whole grain organic bread, raw vegetables, & quality cheeses such as Edam, Gouda, Emmentaler, Sbrinz or Camembert.

Mid-morning - Homemade vegetable juice (carrots, beets with lemon or apple, or greens). Homemade carrot or beet juices are very important cancer-fighters.

Before Lunch (especially serious patients) - Champagne with 1 Tbsp ground Flax seeds in small glass of fruit juice. The champagne helps with absorption of the seeds.

Lunch - Salad plate (tomato, cucumber, lettuce, radish, cabbage, broccoli, and pepper) with homemade Cottage Cheeseand Flax oil mayo dressing (prepared by mixing together 2 Tbsp Flax oil, 2 Tbsp milk, 2 Tbsp Cottage Cheeseand 1 Tbsp lemon juice, add a variety of herbs making the plate most appealing.

Lunch - Main Course Vegetables cooked in water, then flavored with oleolox and herbs possibly with oatmeal, curry etc. Vegetable soups flavored with a little oleolox and nutritional yeast flakes, as side dish for buckwheat, brown rice, millet or potatoes.

Lunch Dessert - Must have 2nd serving of 3 Tbsp. Flax oil and 6 Tbsp. Quark or Cottage Cheese with a little milk and honey, well blended. Add raw fruit, fruit juice, raw nuts, and other flavors you like.

Mid-afternoon - 1 Tbsp. freshly ground Flax seed added to 1 glass of pure fruit juice, homemade.

Late afternoon - Papaya or pineapple juice, 1 glass, with 1 Tbsp Flax seeds freshly ground.

Dinner - Grains alone or grains & beans with vegetables with oleolox, nutritional yeast flakes & spices. Eat buckwheat at least 4 days in a week. Grains & beans combined make a complete protein. Vegetables such as spinach, asparagus, broccoli, & cabbage add nutrition and aid absorption. Dine early.

Late Evening - 1 glass red wine (optional). Go to sleep early - before 10 P.M. if possible.

Prohibitions of Budwig Protocol
- No Sugar, no meat, no eggs, no Butter
- No hydrogenated fat and refined oil
- No soya, corn, peanuts and refined table salt
- No frying, no sautéing, no deep frying
- No preservatives and processed Food
- No microwave, Teflon coated and aluminum cookware
- No cosmetics, chemicals and pesticides
- No foam mattress and pillow.
- No nylon, polyester or acrylic clothing, only cotton, silk and wool is allowed.
- No Cathode ray tube TV and mobile phones
- No leftover food

Elimination or Detoxification

May include (Remember the Mnemonic - M.Sc. Botany)

- **Flax oil massage,**
- **sun therapy,**
- **coffee enema** and
- **soda bicarb bath,** epsom bath, oil pulling, steam bath, sauna bath, liver, colon and kidney cleansing etc.

Energy Therapies (Remember MTV)

- **Meditation**, Meditation, yoga nidra, positive attitude, system change and deep breathing exercises.
- **Tumor contract** – Tell your tumor that if it grows in size, then you may die, and eventually he also will die. So advise him to become microscopic in size. In return you promise to make some changes in your life so that both of you might live long. If he agrees with your proposal, sign a contract with him immediately.
- **Visualization** – is the most important tool to tap into the power of your imagination to help heal cancer. Remain tuned to your healthy and happy future.

Important and must do therapies with Budwig

- Dandelion root 1 Tsp once or twice a day
- Black seed oil as advised by Maria Hurairah
- Bitter apricot kernels - 5 kernels per 5kg of body weight with a Tsp pumpkin seeds
- Essiac tea 30ml to 90ml per day
- Brazil nuts - one nut per day
- Nano curcumin - 1 cap twice or thrice a day
- and Co-enzyme Q-10 - 1 cap once or twice a day
- Nutritional yeast flakes – 1 tablespoon a day

Sauerkraut

Sauerkraut is finely cut cabbage that has been fermented by various lactic acid bacteria. It has a long shelf life and a distinct sour taste, both of which result from the lactic acid that forms when the bacteria ferment the cabbage.

History of Sauerkraut

Sauerkraut originated approximately 2,000 years ago in China. It was known as suan cai, a particular type of "pickled vegetable with sour taste", made by natural fermentation of Napa cabbage or Chinese green. The earliest known history of suan cai is the laborers who built the Wall of China got their nourishment from rice and various types of fermented and pickled vegetables including suan cai. It wasn't until 1,000 years later that Genghis Khan plundered China and brought back this recipe to Europe. The Germans gave it the name "sauerkraut", learned to make this from their native European cabbage.

It soon became a staple for seafaring men. It kept well without refrigeration and the vitamin content found in sauerkraut helped keep the ship's crews scurvy free. The famous ship captain, James Cook, once ordered 25,000 pounds of sauerkraut to outfit two ships.

In World War I and II, the slang word "kraut" was used to refer to sailors and ultimately all German soldiers because of a long history of German ships being outfitted with sauerkraut as part of daily food rations to prevent the onset of scurvy.

Glucosinolates - Trump card in Cancer Treatment

To date, more than 475 studies have proved the role of sauerkraut in cancer prevention and treatment. This is due to the three different types of nutrients. These types are (1) antioxidant, (2) anti-inflammatory, and (3) glucosinolates.

Oxidative stress and chronic inflammation are risk factors for cancer, the antioxidant and anti-inflammatory compounds of sauerkraut provide anti-cancer benefits. But glucosinolates are the trump card with regard to "anti-cancer" benefits. The glucosinolates found in sauerkraut can be converted into isothiocyanate compounds that are cancer preventive for a variety of different cancers.

The body of the cancer patients is always acidic, because the cancer cells constantly ferment the glucose and produce levo-rotating (left rotating) lactic acids. This lactic acid makes our body acidic. You know that cancer cells thrive in acidic environment, but as Warburg discovered, cancer cells cannot survive in an alkaline environment. **It interesting that sauerkraut contains dextro-rotating (right rotating) lactic acids (the good man). This is highly alkaline and neutralizes levo-rotating lactic acids and makes our body alkaline.**

That is why Marcus Porcius Cato the Elder issued a statement - Carcinomas are incurable except with the treatment with Sauerkraut.

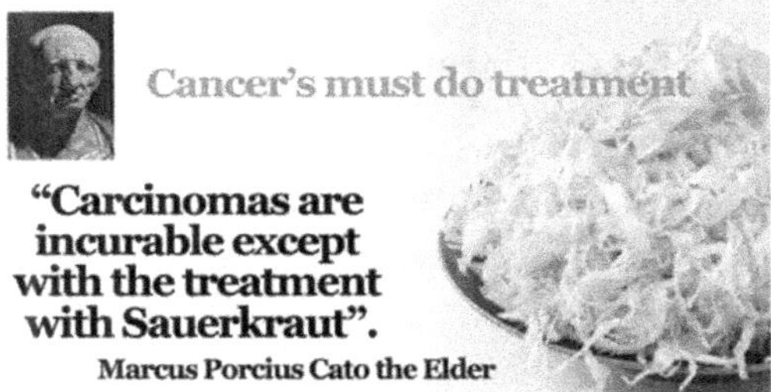

Glucosinolates and their Anti-Cancer Thiocyanates

Indole-3-carbinol (I3C) is a benzopyrrole not an isothiocyanate. It is only formed when isothiocyanates made from glucobrassicin are further broken down into non-sulfur containing compounds.

The isothiocyanates (ITCs) made from cabbage's glucosinolates act to protect us against cancer through a variety of mechanisms. In some cases, they help regulate inflammation by altering the activity of messaging molecules within our body's inflammatory system. In other cases, they improve our body's detoxification system and leave our cells with a smaller toxic load. But the bottom line is decreased risk of cancer from consumption of cabbage and its glucosinolates. We've seen one study, from Poland, showing impressive reduction of breast cancer risk in women consuming large amounts of cabbage.

In this context of glucosinolates, isothiocyanates, and cancer prevention, it is worth noting that one of the I3C (the isothiocyanate made from glucobrassicin) can be further converted in the stomach under healthy acidic conditions to diindolylmethane (DIM), which has also been shown to be a valuable cancer-preventive compound.

Other health benefits of Sauerkraut

Sauerkraut is anti-bacterial, anti-viral, anti-inflammatory, reduces free radicals, boosts immunity, reduces cholesterol, improves blood flow, repairs damaged cells and low in calories.

Promotes Digestion

Cabbage is notable for its high fiber content. Fiber allows a fluent peristaltic movement, encourages regular bowel movements, and eliminates constipation, flatulence, and excess gas. As cabbage ferments, it produces a broad spectrum of bacteria. These probiotics or good bacteria inhabit inside your gut and serve as the first line of defense against pathogens that may enter through the food we eat.

A cup of sauerkraut alone contains approximately 3 billion colony-forming units. Likewise, sauerkraut contains enzymes that help break down nutrients for better absorption. Since probiotics help reduce inflammation and eliminate pathogens that may reside within your digestive tract, probiotics are beneficial for reducing symptoms brought by irritable bowel syndrome.

Boosts The Immune System

Approximately 75% of our immune system relies on our gut integrity. Sauerkraut's probiotics contributes to the immune system by controlling inflammation and inhibiting immune reactions, both of which are the root cause of so many ailments today.

Probiotics help build up a stronger stomach lining to prevent unwanted substances from leaking into your body that may lead to undesirable immune responses. Moreover, maintaining a healthy gut flora is not only vital in the prevention of bacterial manifestation but also for the production of antibodies. A 100 g serving of sauerkraut contains 24% of your recommended dietary allowance for vitamin C, which is one of the most vital elements for our immune system's continued health.

Promotes Heart Health

Fiber is just as vital for heart health as much as for digestion. It helps eliminate fatty deposits within artery walls; hence, reducing the risk for atherosclerosis, heart attacks, strokes, and other heart problems. Moreover, a 100 g serving of sauerkraut contains 6.6-mcg menaquinone that helps reduce heart disease by preventing calcium deposits in the arteries.

Strengthens Bones

As stated above, sour cabbage contains menaquinone or commonly known as vitamin K, which contributes largely in bone health. Vitamin K produces proteins that facilitate bone mineralization and in the absorption of calcium, which is the foundation of strong bones and teeth.

Moreover, sauerkraut's vitamin C content also plays a vital role in bone health since bone building starts with strands of collagen. Crystallized calcium and phosphorus connects to the collagen for bone formation. The amalgamation of minerals and collagen creates a skeletal frame that can withstand impact.

Boosts Mental Health

The brain and digestive system are connected. What you eat can affect your brain and vice versa. Thereby, eating probiotic-rich foods that promotes healthy gut flora can provide positive effects to the brain. Researchers attributed this to the communication via the vagus nerve, which is affected by the good bacteria present in the gut. Furthermore, probiotics have also shown to sharpen memory.

Helps Fight Stress

Probiotics found in sauerkraut have been found to relieve anxiety, depression, and reduce the likelihood of obsessive-compulsive responses. By contributing to the creation of a healthy gut flora, absorption of mood-regulating minerals such as magnesium and zinc are increased to help fight stress and help induce a happy temperament.

Beneficial of Weight Loss

Eating sauerkraut helps curb food cravings. Studies show that people who regularly consume probiotic-rich foods have a lowered risk for obesity. Since sauerkraut is low in calories and high in fiber, it fills your stomach, provides you nutrition, and prevents you from frequent snacking.

Provides Eye and Skincare Benefits

Sauerkraut is rich in vitamin A, an antioxidant that eliminates free radicals from the body and helps prevent premature skin aging. Likewise, vitamin A is vital in eye health and reduces the risk of cataracts and macular degeneration.

Reduces Inflammation and Allergies

Inflammation is the body's response to harmful stimuli. When inflammation occurs, white blood cells are released into the affected tissues to safeguard your body from foreign invaders. However, inflammation is also the root cause of a majority of diseases. Inflammation, when triggered by autoimmunity, causes more harm than good as it enables your body to attack itself. As soon as your body suspects that it is being harmed by a foreign invader, be it food, allergen, poor air quality, or a new type of cosmetic, it attacks it own tissues instead.

Sauerkraut's probiotics help regulate naturally killing cells that controls the body's inflammatory pathways and acts in response accordingly to prevent unnecessary symptoms and puts off chronic diseases.

The Science behind Sauerkraut Lacto-fermentation

Lacto-fermentation is an anaerobic oxidation of carbs present in cabbage, brought about by the Lactobacilli bacteria (lactic acid-producing bacteria LABs). These Lactobacilli reduce the pH, making the environment acidic and unsuitable for the growth of unwanted bacteria. The goal of making sauerkraut is to provide the best environment for Lactobacilli to grow.

Stages of Sauerkraut fermentation

Sauerkraut must go through three specific stages of fermentation.

Stage One

Leuconostoc mesenteroides initiates sauerkraut fermentation. Since Leuconostoc mesenteroides produce carbon dioxide, which effectively replaces the oxygen in the jar, making the environment oxygen-free. When lactic acids reach between 0.25 and 0.3%, Leuconostoc mesenteroides bacteria slow down and die off, but enzymes continue to function. This stage lasts between one and three days, depending on temperature.

Stage Two

Lactobacillus plantarum and Lactobacillus cucumeris continue the ferment until lactic acid level of 1.5-2% is attained. High salt and low temp inhibit these bacteria, so I hope you didn't over-salt your cabbage. This stage continues for 10-30 days, depending on temperature.

Stage Three

Lactobacillus brevis (may be Lactobacillus pentoaceticus also) finish off the ferment. When lactic acid reaches 2-2.5%, they reach their max growth and the ferment is over. This final stage lasts under a week. When no more bubbles appear in the jar, your sauerkraut is ready.

Factors affecting Lacto-fermentation

Although the process is simple, and will complete well if the right amount of salt added, there are some factors that influence how sauerkraut will turn out. These are follows:

Brine level

Bacteria that may spoil sauerkraut will have the upper hand if you have an insufficient level of brine. Too low level of brine allows the undesirable aerobic bacteria and yeasts to grow on the surface. This can cause bad-flavors and discoloration of kraut.

Oxygen

Lactobacillus plantarum, the primary bacteria responsible for Stage Two, works best without oxygen. Presence of oxygen will promote mold formation, allows pink yeasts to grow and could result in soft 'kraut.

Temperature

The ideal temperature to make perfect sauerkraut is 18-24 degrees Celsius. It is very important to maintain this temperature during fermentation period. Temperature also affects enzymes, which are destroyed once the temperature has risen to 45 degrees. Maintain the right temperature.

Salt

Use only iodine-free rock salt at a ratio of about 1 to 3% and mix thoroughly. Much more than this and the Lactobacilli can't thrive, less than this may promote yeast and mold formation.

pH

Since sauerkraut has a pH of 4.6 or lower, it is acidic. The acidic environment will not permit the growth of bacterial spores and thus is resistant to spoilage.

Lactobacilli thrive in an acid environment, but so can molds and yeasts. But always remember that you should keep the oxygen out in order to prevent mold and yeast formation. Yeast and mold both need an oxygen source to thrive.

How To Make Homemade Sauerkraut in a Fido Jar

Ingredients

- 6 Kg green cabbage preferably organic
- Rock salt or Kosher salt
- Caraway seeds one table spoon
- Fido Jar 5 Liter

Instructions

- Peel any unsightly outer leaves off the cabbage and chop off the stem, and then cut in half. Core the cabbage then cut into quarters.
- Using a sharp knife or a slicer/shredder, shred the quarters of cabbage into 1/8 inch strips and place into a huge mixing bowl (make sure you weigh the bowl ahead of time so you can subtract that out to calculate the final weight).
- Weigh the cabbage and calculate how much salt you will need, ideally 1.5%,

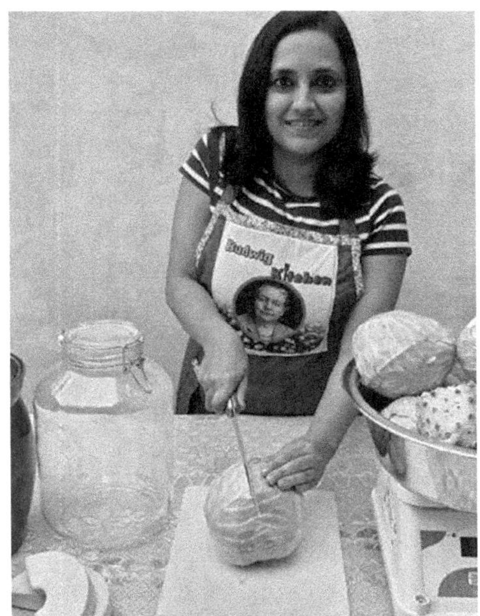

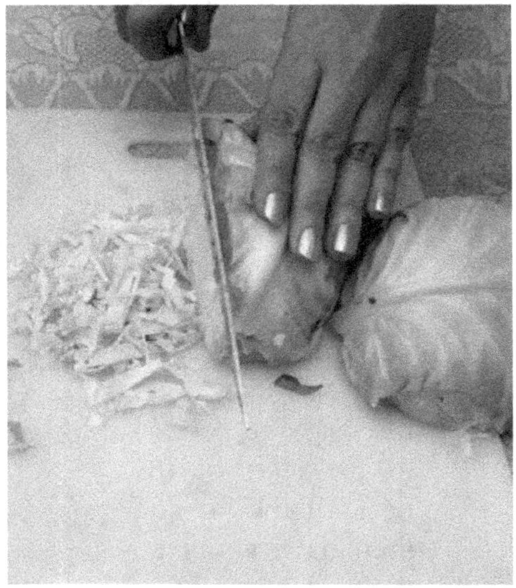

recommended quantity of salt is 1-3%. Measure out the correct amount of salt and put it in to a small bowl. Then add the salt to the cabbage, a little at a time while mixing thoroughly. What you are trying to do here is distribute the salt evenly. You don't want to have pockets that are over salted or under salted.

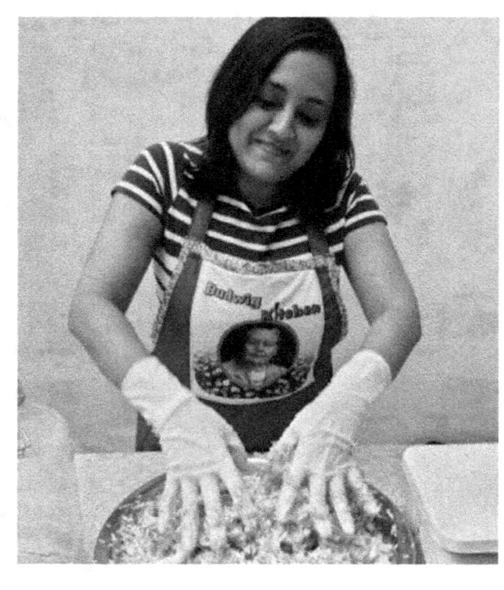

- Once it is fully salted, let sit for about 10 minutes.
- Now comes the fun part. Squeeze, massage, and pound your cabbage for 10 minutes or so. This will cause the cabbage to release its water and create a nice amount of brine.

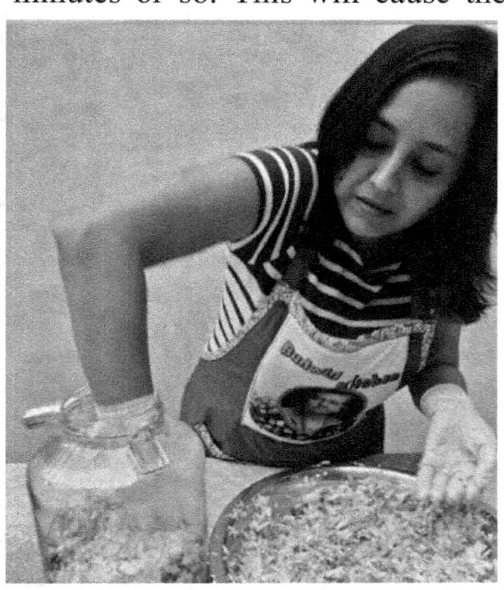

- Now Transfer the cabbage to your Fido jar, smashing it down as you go to pack it really tight. Fill nearly to the top. I like to get the cabbage packed to the start of the neck of the jar and then have about an inch or more of brine covering then maybe an inch of airspace between the brine and the lid.

- Seal the jar and wash off any stray pieces of cabbage or brine that may have soiled the outside during the filling process. Place the jar on a wide rimmed plate and store in a dark closet or cupboard. In the first few days more water might release from the cabbage and the CO_2 build up will likely cause the cabbage to heave 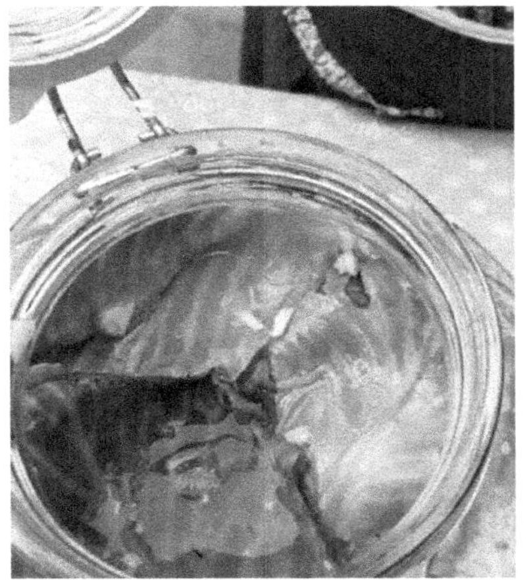 upwards and some brine will push out through the air locked lid. This is all normal and the reason you really need that plate.

- In hot countries like India, it is very difficult to maintain the proper temperature. We have developed a special technique for this issue. You can keep your Fido jar in a water filled clay plant pot. Water will remain cold in the clay pot and thus will maintain the right temperature in the jar. 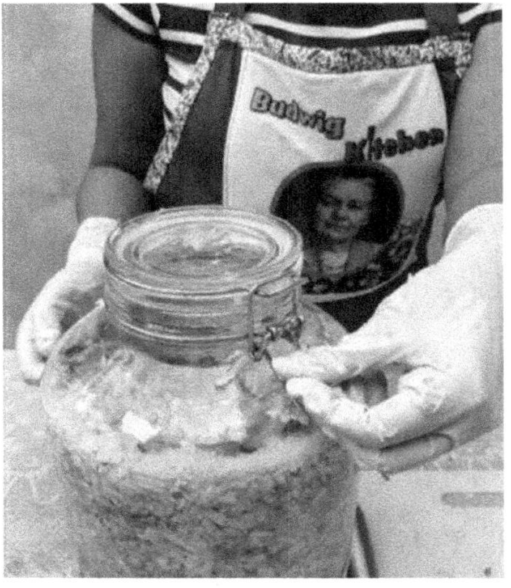

- Wait at least 20 days and up to 8 weeks, one month is ok.

- Enjoy eating your awesome homemade sauerkraut and then store in the fridge.

Joy of the Mountain - Oregano Oil

Wild Oregano (Origanum Vulgare) is a perennial herb that has purple flowers and spade-shaped, olive-green leaves. The whole plant has a strong, peculiar, fragrant, balsamic odour and a warm, bitterish, aromatic taste, both of which properties are preserved even when the herb is dry. The oregano sold as a spice is either Sweet Marjoram (Origanum majorana) or Mexican Sage. Dr. Cass Ingram's book, The Cure is in the Cupboard, describes how oregano can reverse numerous ailments.

There are over 40 oregano species, but the most therapeutically beneficial is the wild oregano or Origanum vulgare that's native to Mediterranean mountains. To obtain oregano oil, the dried flowers and leaves of the plant are harvested when the oil content of the plant is at its highest, and then distilled.

The ancient Greeks and Romans have a profound appreciation for oregano, using it for various medicinal uses. In fact, the name Origanum is derived from two Greek words, oros (mountain) and ganos (joy) – literally means joy of the mountain. It was admired as a symbol of happiness, and it was an ancient tradition to crown brides and grooms with a laurel of oregano.

Composition

Wild Oregano contains 41 antibacterial, 31 anti-inflammatory, 26 antiviral, 26 antifungal, 22 antiseptic, 6 antiparasitic, 28 antioxidant, 6 immunostimulant and 4 COX-2 inhibitor elements.

Carvacrol (a type of phenol) is one of the strongest and most effective multi-spectrum antibiotics known to man, killing 90 different pathogenic microorganisms, such as candida albicans, staphylococcus, E. coli, campylobacter, salmonella, klebsiella, the aspergillus mold, giardia, pseudomonas, and listeria.

Thymol - a natural Cox-2 inhibitor and fungicide with antiseptic properties. It boosts immunity, protects against toxins, and even prevents tissue damage and encourages healing.

Terpenes – powerful antibacterial.

Rosmarinic acid – an antioxidant and helps in treating allergic asthma, cancer and atherosclerosis. It is also a natural antihistamine that reduces fluid buildup and swelling caused by allergy.

Naringin - inhibits the growth of cancer cells and boosts the antioxidants in oregano oil.

Beta-caryophyllin (E-BCP) - this substance inhibits inflammation and is beneficial for osteoporosis, arteriosclerosis, as well as metabolic syndrome.

Nutrients like vitamins A, C, and E, calcium, magnesium, zinc, iron, potassium, manganese, copper, boron, and niacin are also found in oregano oil.

Oregano oil Fights Cancer

Oregano can assist in a holistic cancer treatment. It will not cure cancer alone but in combination with other herbs and therapies, it will boost cancer treatment effectiveness. Carvacrol has the ability to activate the natural anti-inflammatory defense.

Pain Killer

Oregano oil relieves pain as effective as morphine. It even surpassed the ability of conventional drugs to reverse pain and inflammation.

"Less is more" applies to oregano oil

Full strength Oregano oil is too powerful for the internal or even external applications. Dilute it at least 3:1 with any good carrier oil (olive oil or coconut oil). Do spot test before using it in liberal amounts. Dilutions range from 3:1 to 15:1 depending upon the specific use. Do not use in vagina, anus, sensitive skin areas or mucous membranes unless well diluted due to heat sensation.

Normal adult dose is 2-3 drops (diluted 1 part Oregano oil : 3 parts carrier oil), 2-3 times/day. Under the tongue (mix well with saliva before swallowing) or in 4oz. juice, water or mixed into a Tsp. of honey. Drink 6-8 glasses of pure water daily to flush toxins from the blood.

Lothar Hirneise

Great supporter of Budwig Protocol

Eleven years, Lothar Hirneise worked as a trained nurse in the State Psychiatric Hospital in Winnenden. After four years, he took psychoanalysis training. Hirneise was also master in Eastern combat sports and a Kung Fu teacher. He owned a successful sporting goods company, which he sold for a tidy profit in 1986. After a year one of his close friend developed Testicular Cancer. Lothar went in search of information about 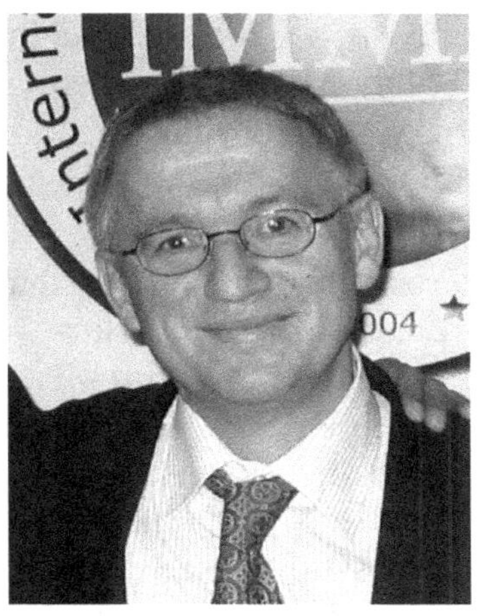 cancer therapies and came across Lynne McTaggart, the founder of the book and magazine "What Doctor's Don't Tell You." Then he was informed that Frank Wiewel, president of the American organization "People Against Cancer", which operates alternative cancer research since 1985, would come to London. So he went to London with his best friend Klaus Pertl to attend this conference for alternative cancer treatments (early 1997). This weekend his friend died. This was the starting point of his intensive quest for potential cancer therapies. He had time and money and read everything he could get his hands on. He nearly went crazy and was severely infected by a virus called Holistic Oncology. He travelled to Bahamas, Mexico, Russia, China, and the United States and all over Europe.

Frank Wiewel advised him to visit Dr. Budwig who lived only 60 km from his home in Germany. Lothar and Klaus Pertl visited Budwig in the spring of 1998, and from the beginning it was an intense relationship that persisted for a very long time.

Over several years he remained in close contact with this great sage of Science. The content of their conversations used to be about fats and electrons. One day she suggested writing a book in which, she could explain her theories again, briefly and concisely. And the Book Cancer - "The Problem And The Solution" was written. Lothar worked very hard in the creation of this great book.

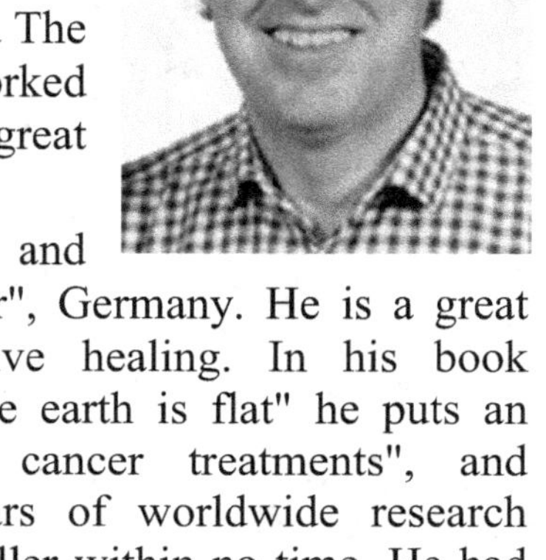

Lothar Hirneise is founder and President of "People Against Cancer", Germany. He is a great researcher and writer on alternative healing. In his book "Chemotherapy cures cancer and the earth is flat" he puts an "Encyclopedia of unconventional cancer treatments", and summarizes the results of his years of worldwide research together. The book became a best seller within no time. He had successfully treated thousands of cancer patients at his center in Germany (3E Zentrum, Buocher Höhe Im Salenhäule 10, D-73630 Remshalden-Buoch Telefon: 07151-98130).

Tumor is not a problem, but a solution

Lothar Hirneise says: "A tumor is the body's solution to some problem in your body. A tumor forms because someone is no longer producing adrenaline, which is needed to break down sugar. An excess of sugar is dangerous, so the body produces tumors. Tumors ferment or burn sugar. Tumors also use a lot of energy - sugar - due to the fast division of cells. Cancer cells function like liver cells, but much more efficiently. So the tumor helps you to get rid of poisons from your body. Without the tumor you would be really ill. That is why you shouldn't immediately operate to remove a tumor. First strengthen and detoxify yourself. If the tumor still continues to grow - which is almost never the case - you can always operate later."

3E Program

He travels a lot in search of finding most successful alternative cancer therapies. In the last few years he has interviewed several hundred final stage so-called survivors, meaning patients who were in the final stage of cancer and who are all healthy again today. Based on his findings he proposed a 3E Program for cancer.

- Eat well
- Eliminate the toxins from the body
- Energy

He noticed that 100% of all survivors, did the energy work. In approximately - say 80% of all patients, 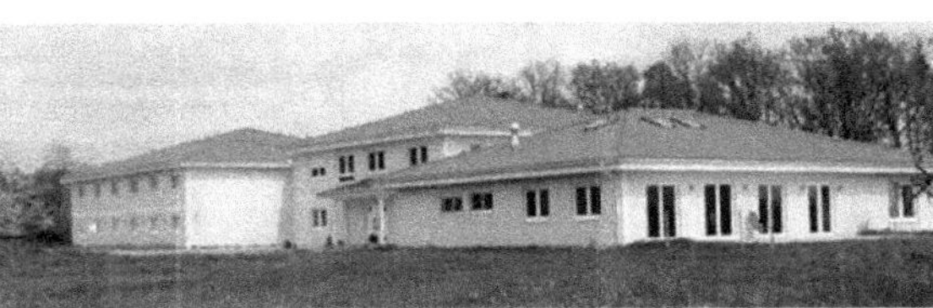 He found a change in diet. And in at least 60% of all patients, took intensive detoxification rituals. This is the basis of his, so much talked about 3E Program for healing cancer.

Diet and Nutrition

He proudly says that he has shaken the hands with hundreds of people, who made extreme dietary change and became well. They are still alive and living a healthy life. If you still believe that Cancer diets are nonsense, go to him, he will prove the opposite. He has interviewed enough patients and knows them personally. Good nutrition naturally means getting energy. He explains that we have three ways and means of getting energy into our bodies.

1. The first is the light. Light is naturally our number one source of energy. He is 100% sure.

2. The second way is organic nutrition. He emphasized strict organic diet; of course, you do not get any energy from a chicken

burger. Rather, when you eat this, you lose some energy, which you have to compensate later.

3. Another possibility which you have is let the energy flow in your body, in your meridians and in your thoughts. Think about the feeling you had last time when you were in love. You felt wonderful; you were on top of the sky. But what did it change? Did your DNA change? Did your cell respiration change? Nothing really changed. The Indians would say your chakras were opened and the energy started to flow freely again. This is the secret, not only to get the energy, but also to let it flow freely. This proves that our thoughts, our mental-spiritual side is too important.

Now back to nutrition. Out of all nutritional therapies of cancer that he had investigated, the Budwig diet is definitely number one. He investigated thousands of patients, Dr. Budwig allowed him to investigate all her cases of the last thirty years, and he concluded that nowhere you find such fantastic cases as with Dr. Budwig, not even remotely. It's amazing. Even patients who were in coma, when received her Oil-Protein Diet, and rubbed so-called electron differential oils (ELDI oils) on the body, did again come out from coma. They were able to eat, walk and live normally today. It is really miraculous. Therefore, her Oil-Protein Diet became the basis of his 3-E Program for cancer patients.

Detoxification

Next important point that he suggests is detoxification. Detoxification actually covers two points.

1. The first is naturally to avoid toxins and poisons e.g. use of cosmetics, toothpaste, etc.

2. And the second point which belongs to detoxification is not to add any toxins in future. The most important point is definitely diet. It doesn't need further explanation. We are ingesting lot of poisons through our diet. Is better not to eat than all this rubbish that one can buy today.

Healthy teeth and gums are phenomenally important. Heat is a very good way to expel poisons. All the parasite cleanses, colon cleansing, ELDI oils, drinking a lot of water is essential. Going out into the sun light, twice daily is very important. You might have listened today that the sun is suddenly bad for you and may cause skin cancer. That is nonsense, forget it. We are all children of the light, we definitely need the light. Even if it's raining and cloudy today go outside. Even if patient is in coma, he must be wheeled out. You should go twice daily into the light. Light increases Vitamin D levels, important for the liver and increases energy levels.

Energy Work

Energy work is the most important point. He divides it into mental and spiritual work. Naturally, you are advised to do meditation and develop positive thinking. You think about life, 'Why do I have cancer and what is the purpose of my life, why am I here on this earth?' and so on. But he focused on something what he called the **SYSTEM CHANGE**. He explains that we all live in Systems. In our marriage, in our house, in our job, etc. Many, many, many of these cancer patients made system jumps. Means that they kicked their husband in the butt and threw him out. They quit their job, they moved, they not only moved their bed, they moved out of their apartment, went to other countries. Quite honestly, I don't know, what should you do? But Lother's experience is that it it's remarkable to what extent people changed their life before they were in a position to get well.

Lothar Hirneise Concludes: "There is no spontaneous remission, there are only people who positively change their life and regained their health that way." (Hirneise, 2005)

Interview of Dr. Johanna Budwig

Lothar Hirneise worked with Dr. Johanna Budwig from 1998 to 2003. He explained that there is much more available to cancer patients than just chemo and irradiation. Mr. Lothar Hirneise conducted this great interview in 1998 (Budwig, Cancer The Problem And The Solution).

Lothar Hirneise: What is your fundamental research?

Dr Johanna Budwig: In 1949, I developed Paper Chromatography of fats with Professor Kaufmann, the director of the Federal Institute for Research on Grain, Potatoes and Fat, and my former doctoral advisor, who was also director of the Pharmaceutical Institute. With this technique for first time I was able to detect fats, fatty acids and lipoproteins directly even in 0.1 ml of blood. I used Co 60 isotopes successfully to produce the first differential reaction for fatty acids, and produced the first direct iodine value via radioiodine. I also developed control of atmosphere in closed system by using gas systems which act as antioxidants. I further developed Coloring, separating effects of fats and fatty acids. I too studied their behavior in blue light, red light with fluorescent dyes.

Using rhodamine red dye, I studied the electrical behavior of the unsaturated fatty acids with their "halo". With this technique I could prove that electron rich highly unsaturated Linoleic and Linolenic fatty acids (Flax oil being richest source) were the mysterious and undiscovered decisive fats in respiratory enzyme function which Otto Warburg could not find. I studied the electromagnetic function of pi-electrons of the linolenic acid in the cell membranes, for all nerve function, secretions, mitosis, as well as cell division. I also examined the synergism of the sulfur containing protein with the Pi-electrons of the highly unsaturated fatty acids and their significance for the formation of the hydrogen bridge between fat and protein, which represent "the only path" for fast and focused Transport of electrons during respiration.

This immediately caused an excitement in scientific community. Everybody thought that it will open new doors in Cancer research. I also proved that Hydrogenated fats, refined oils including all Tran's fatty acids were not having any vital electrons and thus proved as respiratory poisons. We published this research exclusively in many journals including "New Directions in Fat Research".

Lothar Hirneise: What is the prime cause of Cancer?

Dr Johanna Budwig: In 1928 Dr. Otto Warburg proved that all normal cells require oxygen absolutely, but cancer cells can live without oxygen. It is a rule without exception. If you deprive a cell 35% of its oxygen for 48 hours and it would become cancerous. Dr. Otto Warburg has proved it clearly that the root cause of cancer is lack of oxygen in the cells, which creates an acidic state in the human body.

He also discovered that cancer cells are anaerobic i.e. do not breathe oxygen, get the energy by fermentation of glucose producing lactic acid and cannot thrive in the presence of high levels of oxygen. Long back in 1911 Swedish scientist Torsten Thunberg postulated that sulfur containing protein (found in cottage cheese) and some unknown fat is required to attract oxygen in the cell. This fat plays a major role in the cellular respiration. For nearly half century scientists were trying to identify this unknown and mysterious fat but nobody succeeded.

Lothar Hirneise: How did you develop cancer therapy which is called Budwig Protocol?

Dr Johanna Budwig: During my research I found that the blood of seriously ill cancer patients had deficiency of unsaturated essential fats (Linoleic and Linolenic fatty acids), lipoproteins, phosphatides, and hemoglobin. I also noticed that cancer patients had a strange greenish-yellow substance in their blood which is not present in the blood of healthy people. I wanted to develop a healing program for cancer.

So I decided to straight way go for human trials and I enrolled 642 cancer patients from four big hospitals in Münster. I started to give Flax oil and Cottage Cheeseto the cancer patients. After just three months, patients began to improve in health and strength, the yellow green substance in their blood began to disappear, tumors gradually receded and at the same time as the nutrients began to rise. Thus I had a cure 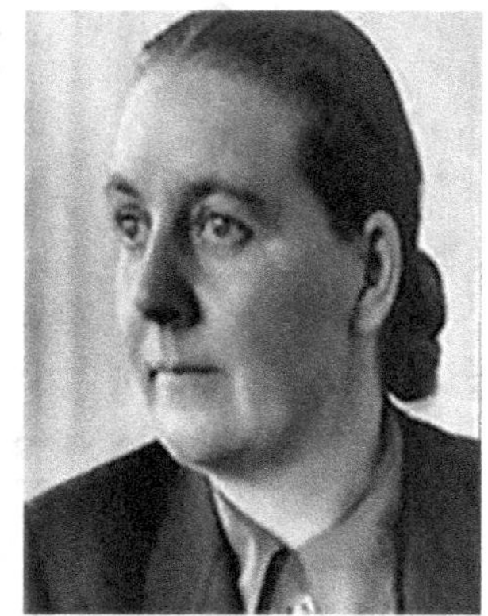 for cancer. It was a great victory and the first milestone in the battle against cancer. My treatment is based on the consumption of Flax seed oil with low fat cottage cheese, raw organic diet, detoxification, mild exercise, Flax oil massage and the healing powers of the sun. I have treated approx. 2500 cancer patients during last few decades. Prof. Halme of surgery clinic in Helsinki used to keep records of my patients. According to him my success was over 90% and this too was achieved in cases where conventional Oncology failed.

Lothar Hirneise: Can you tell us more about the unsaturated fatty acids and their net-like connections?

Dr. Johanna Budwig: Fatty acid is a carboxylic acid having unbranched chain of 4 to 28 carbons. The saturated fatty acids have primarily short carbon chains. In butter, coconut fat, goat fat and sheep fat the fatty acids consists of 4, 6, 8, 10 or 12 carbons. These fats are saturated, however they can also easily metabolize if the essential fatty acids are present. The unsaturated vital fatty acids really start with the chain with 18 carbon compounds. There are also fatty acids with up to 30 carbons. Fatty acids with 18 carbons, like in Flax oil with the higher level of unsaturation, are more important for human beings, particularly for the brain functions of man. Linoleic acid rich in electrons is considered vital. There is particularly high amount of energy in this double double bonds of the linoleic acid.

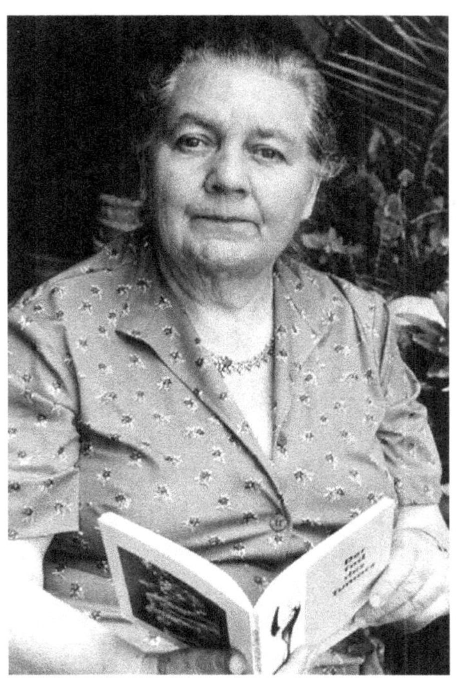

This energy wanders and is not fixed in place while in a chemical compound, such as with table salt the energy is fixed. This energy, wandering between electrons and the positively charged protein with sulfur groups is an alternating association process in the electromagnetic field. This is very important. Perhaps you are familiar with the painting of Michelangelo, where God creates Adam (two fingers pointing to each other, however they do not touch). This is quantum physics, here the fingers do not touch. The physicists who I know, Max Planck, or Albert Einstein, or Dessauer all represent the view that man is created by God in His image. You see in being together as human beings there is certainly also a connection without directly touching the other person. The dipolarity with a single double bond in olive oil is weaker than it is in sunflower seed oil, which is has two double bonds. This double double bond is considered to be vital for man. However if the same chain length of 18 carbons has three unsaturated fatty acid double bonds, then the electrical energy is as strong as a magnet. This electronic energy is negatively charged. The positively charged sulfur groups of the protein adhere in the unsaturated bonds where the electrons are and that is where they insert their sulfur-containing compounds.

This produces the lipoproteins. The life process is sustained in the interplay between the positively-charged particles and negatively-charged particles. In this process there is no connection, and this is our life element. If radical damage occurs at this point through fatty acids that has lost electron energy, but rather are cross-linked like a net, then the dipolarity can no longer work actively in this net. This is the deadly effect of free radicals, because instead of the chains with the electron clouds they interlace like a net without electron clouds, indeed with unsaturated bonds, but without dipolarity. I quickly knew that the triple unsaturated fatty acids, which were called linolenic acid, and which no one had isolated before me, had 18 carbons and that they did not always carry their double bonds at the same point. They have such a strong electronic energy compared to the heavier matter in the 18-link fatty acid chains, that biologically this energy is far greater than it is with the next arachidonic acid with 20 links. The highest electron collection is with the combination of linoleic-linolenic fatty acids in Flax oil. The linolenic acid as conjugated (interaction of neighboring double bonds in the molecule that are separated by a single bond) fatty acid is even more effective and is even more strongly interplay with linoleic acid as it is present in the Flax oil for oxygen absorption. This was relatively easy for me to verify in my experiments. I would like to emphasize this. The combination of double unsaturated linoleic acid with triple unsaturated linolenic acid is particularly well-combined in Flax seed.

Lothar Hirneise: Is it this energy that heals cancer?

Dr. Johanna Budwig: Yes, this energy is now movable and it is easily released. It is precisely this energy that heals cancer, or does not even allow it to occur. If this vital element is present then no tumor can exist. This vital element is a deciding factor in the immune system. There is no effective factor in the immune system other than the essential fatty acids.

Lothar Hirneise: What is an electron cloud?

Dr Johanna Budwig: If the enhancement of electronic energy is always higher through absorption of sun photons in the unsaturated fatty acids e.g. in linolenic fatty acids, then the power of the electrons is so high in the dipolarity between gravity and electrons, that they lifts off of the heavy mass and floats like a cloud hence I called them electron cloud.

Lothar Hirneise: What is the significance of the cloud?

Dr. Johanna Budwig: No life form has as much energy to store the electrons and photons as doe's man. The electronic energy stored particularly in the vital, highly unsaturated fatty acids, is very strong life element for man. Man cannot live without them. If oils are treated with heat and harsh chemicals (during refining and hydrogenation process to increase their shelf life) then the wealth of vital electronic energy is destroyed and Tran's fats are formed with net like connections. They are no longer vital fats with 18 carbons, but rather they form cross-links between the fatty acids like a large net, and are highly damaging to our body, do not adhere with proteins, do not attract oxygen and act like a free radicals. I repeat because it is so important: I have detected particles in oils treated with steam, which indeed have a positive iodine value, but which are highly toxic for man.

Lothar Hirneise: So you preach against these toxic hydrogenated and refined oils?

Saturated Fat   Unsaturated Fat   Trans fat

Dr. Johanna Budwig: I am completely against using these "pseudo" fats - "hydrogenated" or "partially hydrogenated". These are the biggest enemy of mankind. I had scientific proofs. The heart rejects these fats and they are deposited as inorganic fat on the heart muscle itself. They end up blocking circulation, damage heart action, inhibit cell renewal and impede the free flow of blood and lymph fluids.

But it was highly profitable business for multinationals. When I preached against these fats, they stood against me, first they tried to bribe me and when I refused they filed many fake court cases against me. I was working for humanity and had scientific proof. I was like rock of Gibraltar in my decision; I fought and won all the cases ultimately.

Lothar Hirneise: What is your view point about surgery for tumors?

Dr. Johanna Budwig: I am totally against radiation and chemo; I also reject hormonal treatment. Surgery must be considered individually. I am not a proponent of quickly making artificial anus. Conventional oncology no longer does justice to the cancer patients.

Lothar Hirneise: You also studied medicine at the age of 47 years.

Dr. Johanna Budwig: (smiling) 😊 Yes handsome! That's right, my opponents were accusing me that how can I treat cancer patients without a doctors degree. This thing pinched me, so in 1955, I joined medical school in Göttingen. There I was using my therapy very successfully in various clinics. I still remember the time I was working late one night in Göttingen, a woman came to me, with her small child whose arm was supposed to be amputated due to a tumor. I treated her and soon the subject of amputation was dismissed and the child quickly did very well.

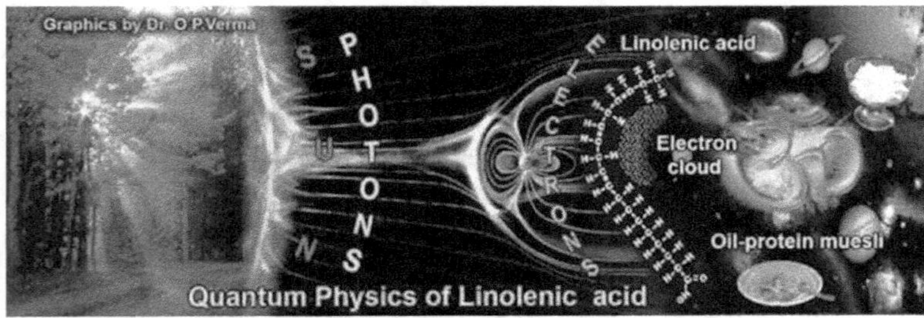

Because I was still a medical student at this time, I was summoned to appear before the Municipal Court due to a petition that I should be prohibited from studying medicine. I explained the truth in the court. The judge rejected the case and said, "You have done a good job, Budwig. In my area of jurisdiction nothing will happen to you. If it does there will be a scandal in the scientific community."

Lothar Hirneise: What do you recommend for prevention of cancer?

Dr. Johanna Budwig: Consume only Flax oil as oil. I reject frozen and preserved meat. Fresh meat is OK. No frozen food and no bakery products. No Tran's fats. Eat organic diet. Oleolox should be used as butter. Prepare fruit juices yourself. Cheese and potatoes are OK. Also the electromagnetic environment (e.g. microwave and mobile phones etc.) in which we live is very important. I reject synthetic textiles and foam mattresses because they steal lot of electrons from you. A lot of wood in home construction and woolen or silk carpets are also important. Wear gemstones, they also have good biological radiation. Books could be written on gemstones. The environment and living conditions must be as biological (organic & natural) as possible. Regular sleep is very important.

Sun, Photons and Electrons

Sun, photons, electrons - What are they?

Sun rays reach the earth as an inexhaustible source of energy. The sources of power in mineral oil, coal, green plant-foods and fruits are based on the energy supplied by the sun's radiation. Light is the fastest traveler from star to star. There is nothing that travels faster than light. Light speeds along with time. Physicists emphasize that the photon, the quantum, the smallest component of the sun's rays is eternal. It is truly a life element. Life is impossible without the photon.

The photon is always in motion. Nothing can ever halt its motion. The photon is full of colors and can change its color, its frequency, when present in large numbers. The photon - acknowledged to be the purest form of energy, the purest wave, always in motion—can unite with a second photon, when it is in resonance with the other, to form a "short-lived particle." This particle, known as "O" particle, can break up into two photons again, without mass, as a pure wave in motion. This is the basis for the wonderful back and forth movement between light and matter. This photon can never be pinned down to one location. This is the foundation for the Theory of Relativity. The photon gave rise to Max Planck's and Einstein's formation of the quantum theory which is of such significance today.

Electrons

Electrons are a smallest particles of matter and are in continual movements. They vibrate continually on their own wavelength. They have their own frequency, like radio receivers which are set at a certain wavelength. The electron orbits in matter around a nucleus. The heavy matter in the nucleus (proton) is charged with positive electricity. In contrast to this, the electron carries a negative charge. The positively charged nucleus and the negatively charged electron attract each other by means of their electrical opposition. But the electron, always in motion, never approaches the nucleus close enough to be drawn out of its own orbit. It maintains a certain freedom of movement within its prescribed orbit.

The electron loves photons. It attracts photons by its magnetic field. When an electrical charge moves, it always produces a magnetic field. The moving photon also has a magnetic field. Both fields, the magnetic field of the electrons and the magnetic field of the photons attract each other when the wavelengths are in tune. The wave length of the photon—which the photon can change—must fit into the wavelength of the orbiting electron so that the orbit maintains a complete wavelength. This feature is extremely interesting in terms of its physical, biological and even philosophical consequences. Matter always has its own vibration, and so, of course, does the living body. The absorption of energy must correspond to one's own wavelength.

Sunbeams are very much in harmony with human. It is no coincidence that we love the sun. The quantum biologists say that the resonance in our body is so strongly tuned to the sun's energy that: There is nothing else on earth with a higher concentration of photons of the sun's energy than man. This concentration of the sun's energy with their highly suitable wavelengths is improved when we eat electron-rich food. The electrons attract the electromagnetic waves of sunbeams. Flax seed oil contain high amount of electrons which are on the wavelength of the sun's energy. Scientifically, these oils are even known as electron-rich essential highly unsaturated fats. *The famous Quantum Physicist Dessauer writes: If it were possible to increase' the concentration of solar electrons tenfold in this electron-rich unsaturated fats, then man would be able to live 10,000 years.*

The sun's energy and man as an antenna

Almost everyone knows what an antenna is. The marvelous science of Maxwell, the physicist, concerning electro-magnetic waves today are well-researched and of practical use. Famous examples are telegraphy, radio, television, microwave oven, cell phones and various applications of high-frequency technology in the manufacturing of electromagnets, the atom bomb and research into nuclear power as a source of energy. Maxwell was able to show that an electric current flowing in an electrically conductive matter produces a magnetic field. Also electrically conductive matter which is moved within a magnet's field, will produce a current. When an atomic particle, such as an electron, is accelerated by an electric field, this produces electric and magnetic fields, which travel at right angles to each other, produces electromagnetic wave. These fundamental, elementary laws can also be applied to biological processes.

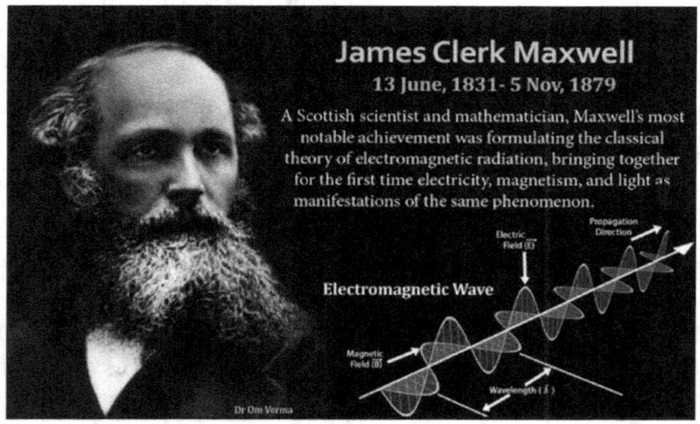

When the sun shines on the leafy canopy of a tree and is absorbed through photosynthesis, this causes movement in the electrical charge of the electrons. A magnetic field is also brought about when the water in trees rises. When we, with our wealth of electrons and conductive living substance, move through the electro-magnetic field of a forest, then a charging with solar electrons takes place in us. When our blood circulates, there is a movement of the electrical charge in the magnetic fields (for example, on the surface lipids of red blood corpuscles), which then causes much induction and re-induction of energy.

With each heartbeat, a dose of the body's own electron-rich, highly unsaturated fats from the lymph system, together with lymph fluid, goes into the blood vessels and thereby into the heart. This constantly stimulates and strengthens the electro-motoric functioning of the heart; Even the movement of the bloodstream is connected with radiation of electromagnetic waves-in accordance with the fundamental law of nature which governs electro-magnetic waves. This Transmitter within humans is always in action.

This Transmitter is also observed in neurons. The cylindrical structure of our nerves with the different layers and ganglions, with the difference in electrical potential between the neurons and dendrites, immediately supplies the picture of how strongly an electric current in a magnetic field leads to the emitting of electromagnetic waves. When I think a positive thought about another person, this involves the emitting of electromagnetic waves. The reception of thought also depends on the wavelength to which the receiver is tuned. There are amplifiers, as well as Transmitters that interfere. This encompasses a whole host of situations that are known under different names such as telepathy, hypnosis, mental telepathy, and many others.

Among Nordic peoples, it is known that the isolated native inhabitants use a tree to amplify thought Transmission, for example, to inform the husband who had gone to town, that he should bring back some salt. Bismark described how, during periods of trouble or pressure, he found relaxation by putting his arms around a tree and leaning his forehead against the trunk. In both cases, it involves electromagnetic waves that behave in accord with Maxwell's mathematical equations.

Fats Syndrome

The special relationship between photons, electrons and Essential Fats (EFAs) described by Dr. Budwig is due to the amazing molecular structures of LA (cis-linoleic acid) and ALA (cis-linolenic acid). The cis-configuration allows de-localized electron clouds (pi-electrons) to collect in the bend produced on the chain. The resulting electrostatic force enables the EFAs to capture oxygen molecules and hold proteins within cell membranes. Like static electricity in a capacitor these charges can produce measurable bioelectric currents essential to nerve, muscle, heart and membrane functions. EFAs are extremely important to the body's overall energy exchange potential — the flow of life force.

Let us concentrate on the actual fats syndrome with its effects on the brain and nerve functions, the organs of the senses, the secretion of mucous, the functioning of the stomach and intestinal tract, liver, gall bladder and kidneys, the lymph and blood vessels, the skin, respiration, the immunity system, the fertilization processes and sexuality. All of these systems and processes of the human being are very much connected with electron-rich highly unsaturated fats, as receivers, amplifiers and Transmitters of electro-magnetic waves, and as supervisor of the vital functions. *The famous Quantum Physicist Dessauer writes: If it were possible to increase the concentration of solar electrons tenfold in this electron-rich unsaturated fat molecule, then man would be able to live 10,000 years.*

Anti-Mensch

Physicists interpret from mathematical formulae that man, with his wealth of electrons, is directed forward in time, which conceals within him the greatest potential to attract the sun's energy, and is directed against entropy. By means of these mathematical formulae, applied to Physics, and by reversing time, the mirror image of human beings is coined—the "Anti-Mensch", lacking electrons, lacks power and strength and directed into the past. It increases the occurrence of cancer. His thought processes, too—is paralyzed, because the element of life, the sun-attuned electrons, is missing.

The process by which x-rays, gamma rays, atom bombs or cobalt rays are set in motion is also equally directed toward the development of the "Anti-Mensch". The electronic structure of the vital functions is destroyed by such rays. According to Feynman's "World Line Diagram" and modern theory of relativity, time and space have been given a relationship in a formula. The "Anti-Mensch" is directed into the past. Human's body tissues with its interplay between solar energy photons and large number of electrons, with its concentration of photons in life's activities and in the dynamics of the vital functions, are directed into the future.

But, when people began to hydrogenate the oils to increase their shelf-life; no-one thought about the consequences of this. In this process these vitally important electrons were destroyed. During hydrogenation, vegetable oils are reacted with hydrogen gas at high temperature. A nickel is used to speed up the reaction and unsaturated fats are hardened. This negative aspect concerning the development of the "Anti-Mensch" is in accordance with Feynman's "World Line Diagram". I emphasize that it means the fats and oils which have had their electron structure destroyed serve, within time and space, to promote the development of the "Anti-Mensch".

The electrons as resonance system

The electrons in our food serve as the resonance system for the sun's energy. Their electro-magnetic field attracts the photons in sunlight. The physicist cannot imagine life without these active and vital photons. These photons, which are in resonance with the electrons in seed oils, are focused on the same wavelength as the sun's energy, serve the life element. This interplay of solar energy photons and the electrons in seed oils governs all the vital functions. Fats are the dominant factor for all the vital functions, according to Ivar Bang.

The electrons of highly unsaturated fats from seed oils, which are on the same wavelength as sunlight, are capable of drawing solar energy and storing it, then, upon demand, of activating it as the purest energy in the form of the electrons clouds, and making it available for the vital functions. All the vital functions are closely connected with membrane function.

The exchange of electrons, the distribution of energy in the whole organism is dependent on these membrane functions — in the nerve pathways, the brain, in every organ, the liver, gall bladder and pancreas in the stomach's mucous membrane and in the kidneys and intestinal tract. The controlling functions of these membranes with their electro-motoric power, is felt everywhere. This is also true for the respiratory functions, and in oxygen absorption and utilization. It also applies to cell division — to all normal growth processes. It is true for the catabolism of substance in the elimination processes taking place by way of the kidneys, intestinal tract and also for the growth of hair and nails, as well as for the development of young life in the womb. Most significant point is that it is this electronic energy that heals cancer. This turning point in the field of proven successful cancer therapy is only one aspect of much bigger picture of the Quantum Biology. A lot of mysteries and miracles have yet to be discovered by doing research in Quantum Biology.

How can we once more reach the peak of human development?

Freeing you from the influences and effects of radiation and from environmental factors which promote development into the "Anti-Mensch", seem important. These goals, set by the individual who chooses, or by the state and food industries with their organization and planning, should be to see that the food we eat consists of electron-rich nutrition. An electron-rich food intake which supplies us with the resonance system for the sun's energy, must once more achieve priority. Such food, as the life element, promotes our sun-attuned energy. This in turn promotes our development, in space and time, into the future. The entire self can then grow and continue to develop further until, in accordance with the laws of nature which govern light and life, the highest level of our being is achieved. *(Excerpted from Dr Johanna Budwig's book "Flax Oil as a True Aid Against Arthritis, Heart Infarction, Cancer and Other Diseases.")*

Daylight

Dr Budwig focused upon the importance of daylight to our health. It is not enough to absorb electrons only through food, but it is important that we feed ourselves so that our cells are able to absorb and process the light coming from the sun. The more sickly someone is, the sooner he is "in the house", which can be a catastrophic mistake. Especially when people are already in a very late stage of the illness, they are often not able to eat enough and good advice is then very difficult. In such cases, Dr Budwig advises to concentrate on the following three points:

- ELDI oils as whole body rubbings and if possible as enemas
- Only freshly squeezed juices and distributed as food throughout the day if possible the breakfast muesli in different variants
- Stay outside as much as possible

You will experience me to explain what to do next. I have been able to see in my life how Dr Budwig's theoretical considerations work when put to practice, if indeed, if they are consistently carried out. If you could experience such a case yourself, and how quickly it can be better for a seriously ill person, you can see Dr Budwig's words in a very different light.

But other great researchers had also dealt with the subject of light long before Dr Budwig. For example, the anthroposophist Rudolf Steiner wrote, about 50 years earlier that there is a fundamental being of our material existence of the earth, of which all materiality has come only through condensation. Every matter on earth is condensed light! There is nothing in material existence, which is something else than condensed light in some form. Wherever you go and feel matter, you have condensed light everywhere. Compressed light. Matter is light by its very nature. In as much as a man is a material being, he is woven of light. Rudolf Steiner and Dr Budwig have pointed out in their writings over and over again the importance of light and that we humans are now heliotropes, which need light and use light. But I have nowhere else than with Dr Budwig so clearly and understandably read, WHY this is and above all, how the charging of the life battery works and / or what importance mainly the linolenic acid or electron clouds play. Because it is so important, I would like to repeat here again: The sicklier someone is, the more he should be in the open." (Oil-Protein Diet by Lothar Hirneise)

Visualization - Path to wellness

The visualization is perhaps the most important tool to tap into the power of your imagination to help heal cancer, manage problems or rather achieve anything in your life. Learning to direct and control images in your mind can help you to relax. This may help to

- Relieve stress
- Control some of the symptoms caused by your cancer or cancer treatments
- Boost your immune system to help your body fight off infections and promote healing

Past   Future

Whatever you see around yourself is just a vision in the beginning, For example the cup of coffee you are holding in your hands or the house in which you live today did not exist in the past. Not very long ago there was a thought in your mind that you want to construct a dream house for living. Then you made construction designs and all sort of workup. Our whole life runs on the rails of time and never turns back. This is our time line.

First of all understand that everything around us is just a thought, energy or a wave. It is significant to understand this. Then only you will believe that energy can be converted in to a matter. Just imagine that a hypnotist puts a coin on your palm and makes you believe that it is hot. You feel burning in your palm. You may even have blisters on your palm. Here the temperature of coin just changed through only.

If you have believed that certain thought can change the condition of your body within seconds. Then why not a good thought can heal your tumor. In many studies Visualization trainer Carl Simomton has proved that cancer patients live twice if they follow visualization technique systematically.

Lothar Hirneise, the student of Dr. Johanna Budwig, respects Carl's research too much except a few points. Simomton teaches his cancer patients to visualize that their white cells are attacking cancer cells and killing them. Lothar is against this school of thought. Because in this situation patient focuses on his tumor. But Lothar says that main problem is something else, tumor problem is secondary. Secondly patient thinks of a war with a cancer cell, while Lothar believes that cancer patient needs balance and harmony rather than thinking of a war.

Lothar has interviewed hundreds of cancer survivors and came to the conclusion that cancer patient avoids direct confrontation with his tumor, but wants to remain busy in dealing with healthy and happy future. Though every patient has different approach, but end is same, creating a happy future. Lothar admits that visualization is the single most important therapy in his so much talked about 3E Program. After all if we will not create a healthy future for us then who else will do.

Please, review your time line again and compare it with thought-matter line. You will notice that both lines travel in the same direction and never turn back. You can never change the direction of any line. So start now and create your own happy future yourself.

Thought   Matter

————————————————————————————➤

Past   Future

————————————————————————————➤

I am going to discuss Lothar's technique in detail, which he learned from Europe's famous Visualization trainers Jack Black from Glasgow. Jack has taught his Mind Store System to 50,000 people in last few years. He is consultant of many celebrities and several companies. Lothar recommends that every cancer patient should attend seminars of Jack Black or Klaus Partl. Klaus Partl is right hand of Lothar Hirneise and teaches visualization at his 3E Center in Germany.

Initially Cancer patient thinks that the most important job is to destroy tumor. If he gets rid of tumor then he can plan to take some holistic treatments e.g. visualization. This is very bad decision. It is very important to follow visualization techniques as a part of your tumor destruction program.

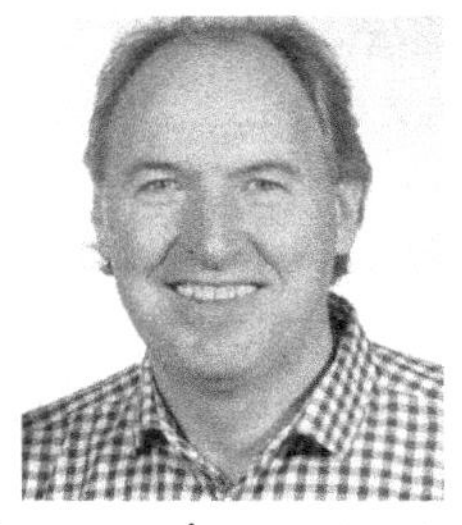

But How does it work? This word HOW is very important, because it usually prevents us to take right decisions. At this moment don't try to think how visualization shall work, how it is going to destroy your tumor. Time being I just say that try to trust us that it actually works.

In short I just say that you learn how to make your future healthy and cheerful, do not focus on present and past. Lothar says that if you know your past, it is easier to change your future. But your main focus should be to create happy future.

Your dream house where you heal your cancer

To give positive impact on your body and mind, it is very important that you become completely relaxed before you start thinking and visualizing. Relaxation or rather achieving alpha stage is the first step. Alpha means relaxed stage (7-14 hertz waves) of your mind. You can relate it with the alpha waves of an EEG tracing. Then there are beta, theta and delta waves. To reach this state there are many techniques or meditations. Some books and CDs are also available. Even listening classical music, meditation or mild yoga can relax you.

When you achieve deep relaxation, start thinking and visualizing. You start it by walking slowly along the right bank of a river. After a short distance you turn towards right. You see blue sky and green meadows. There are lot of trees and a very beautiful house with red terrace. (can imagine your dream house)

Now you enter this house. First room is a beautiful bathroom with a shower. You start taking shower. It washes out all your negativity, toxins and dis-eased cells. After taking shower you sit under the sun, the sunshine dries and fills you with energy within a couple of moments.

Now you go to screen room. On the blank wall of this room there are 3 big LCD monitors. You can relax on the comfortable sofa. You can control these screens with a remote control. On the side table of sofa there also lays a universal DVD recorder. Left screen shows your future, right one the past and the central screen shows your present.

Switch on the central screen, it shows your present sickness. Accept that many people suffered from this illness, you are not alone. Now switch on the right screen to see if you suffered from similar illness in the past. And if you suffered, then how did you treat it. Usually we don't find solution of current problems in the past. Now you minimize and freeze the past screen with remote control. Also, minimize and freeze the present screen.

Now relax and switch on future screen and try to find a solution to your problems. Now visualize a situation where you look perfectly healthy and your tumor has already dissolved. For example if you suffer from bone sarcoma in your thigh and can't even walk due to this illness; you may imagine that you are skiing in Switzerland. Feel the snow peaks, cold breezes, your friend's laughter, your own respiration sounds. Magnify these images, even increase brightness and contrast, and feel the reflection of these images on your body.

You may go to screen room daily, whenever you get time and see yourself skiing. Now you need not to view central and right screen any more. Directly start left screen, our next job is to record this skiing video on universal DVD recorder. The universal DVD recorder will relay this broadcast to the whole world. Your all nears and dears will know about your dream and start helping you to achieve this. To conclude the session, come out of the house and return to the river. Count up to seven and slowly open your eyes. Take a deep breath. This ends your visualization. Always keep in mind that the end should always be happy for everybody; nobody should be harmed any way.

Renovate your dream house if needed

You can construct some extra rooms in this house, if there is a need. For example you can make a small room for rest and relaxation. If you have some pain then you go to this room to relax for a while. You can also make a meeting room. You can invite here some important person to discuss your problem. For example you can call Dr. Johanna Budwig. You can sit with her, discuss and ask her opinion to solve your problem.

You can also invite your friends and close relatives to celebrate your successful skiing expedition. Imagine you are standing on the dice and narrating your experiences and everybody is clapping. The main essence of the story is that in the end people see you are healthy and cheerful. So that they also help you achieve your healthy and happy future. One question is very frequently asked is that how many times you should go to this house. Lothar says that there is no fixed rule but whenever you get time you should visit this house, may be twice a day. If the problem is serious then it is better you go there several times a day.

Visualization wonderfully brings positive changes in your health. It costs nothing but works 100%. You can use this treatment to heal your cancer, make your life happy and cheerful or even to just become a millionaire (Hirneise, 530).

Tumor contract

Tumor contract is an agreement between you and your tumor so that both of you may lead a healthy and longer life. It really looks funny, to make an agreement with your tumor. But you might have done lot of things in your life even crazier than this.

When you are told that you have a cancer, you become worried and depressed. You develop fear that you are going to die very soon. You want to abuse your tumor. But don't do that. Better you talk to him peacefully; after all your tumor is a part of your body. Explain him that if he grows like this, you may die one day and then he also dies. Explain this thing very clearly to him. I am sure that he too shall be frightened after listening this. He may ask you to find a solution for this problem. Tell him that both of you can only survive if he becomes microscopically so small that he is no longer detected in any scan or investigation. To achieve this you also have to make some changes in your life. If he agrees, prepare the agreement documents and get signed immediately. In the preface of the contract mention the changes you are going to make in your life.

Please take this contract very seriously and follow it 100%. This is very important; otherwise tumor will not keep his part of the contract. Mr. Lothar Hirneise has got extremely positive experiences with this therapy, and the more he work with it, the better he understands the ingenious processes that occur in a person when he makes such a contract with his own cells. .

I just want to explain to you that tumors are not a second ego. They are a part of you, but for some reason, they have been severely neglected. It is a kind of situation in a large family, where one member does not get enough attention and he does a mischief to draw attention of other members. The tumor does the same thing. He creates its own attention by growing rapidly.

Below I am giving a sample contract which you should just fill out, after you have completely read this chapter. Keep this contract under your mattress and sleep over it at least a few nights. Then you can keep it in your cupboard. This contract gives very good results if you take it seriously (Hirneise, 517).

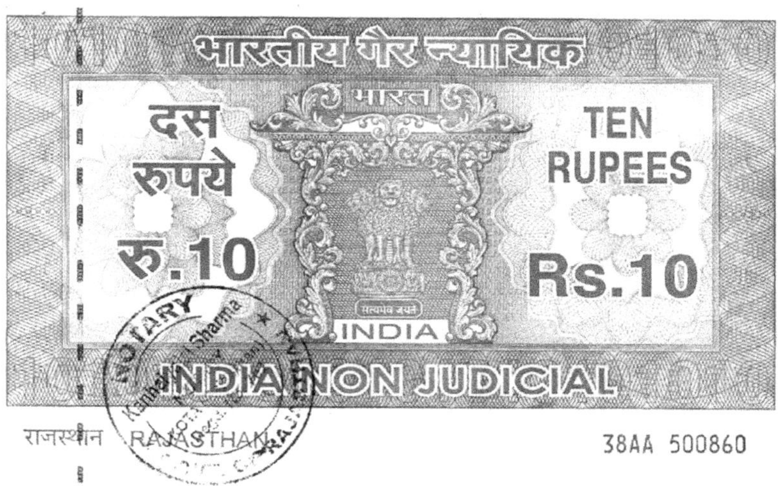

Tumor Contract

The following is agreed between

Tumor and all distant metastases or cell changes

(The TUMOR)

And

(yourself CONTRACT PARTNER)

Preface

Both parties obligate themselves to conclude a contract which describes in detail what each party will undertake so that they jointly can live longer in health and happiness.

(1)

TUMOR agrees that it will become microscopically so small that CONTRACT PARTNER will no longer be consciously aware of it, or that other disorders are not caused by TUMOR.

(2)

CONTRACT PARTNER obligates himself to execute the following changes in his life:

....
....
....
....
....
....
....
....
....
....
....
....
....
....
....
....
....
....
....
....
....

Signature
CONTRACT PARTNER

(3)

Severability Clause

Should compliance with for one or another of the provisions of this contract become impossible - for any reasons beyond the control of either party - then also the contract will still remain in action and both parties will look for a solution which most nearly approaches the original intention. This contract will be analyzed after 3 months at the latest, and it will be extended for an additional 3 months. These extensions will take place for at least 10 years but cannot be cancelled by either partner.

Signature   Signature
TUMOR   CONTRACT PARTNER

Place
Date

Evidence (1) Name:
              Address:

Evidence (2) Name:
              Address:

Unresolved trauma or shock

an important cause of cancer

Germany's famous Surgeon and Cancer Specialist Dr. Ryke Geerd Hamer was studying psychological aspects of cancer and treatment since ten years. He examined and tested over 40,000 cancer patients. He was amazed that why cancer of an organ does not spread to neighboring organ, e.g. he never saw cancer cervix and cancer uterus in a same patient. He also noted that each of his cancer patients suffered a psychological stress or shock during last 3 to 5 years prior to diagnosis and he was not able to come out of that trauma (Puna Wai Ora Mind-Body Cancer Clinic , 2006-2014).

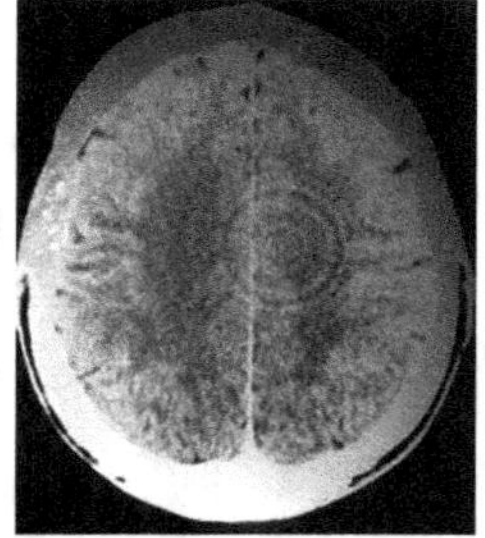

Each patient of Dr. Hamer also underwent CT scan of the head and in all cases he noticed some dark shadow or concentric circles somewhere in the brain. These dark circles would be in exactly the same place in the brain for the particular types of cancer. There was also a 100% correlation between the location of dark circles in the brain, the location of the cancer in the body and the specific type of unresolved conflict. It was very astonishing. Opponent radiologists said that the spots in the CT scans were machine errors (Artifacts). But Siemens Company which made the machine also admitted that these spots are not Artifacts (Hamer).

Thus Dr. Hamer concludes that when we are in a stressful conflict which is not resolved, the emotional reflex center in the brain which corresponds to the experienced emotion (e.g. anger, frustration, grief) will slowly break down. Each of these emotional centers are also connected to a specific organ. When a centre breaks down, it starts sending wrong signals to the organ it controls, resulting in the formation of deformed cells in the tissues, cancer cells. He also suggests that metastasis is not the SAME cancer spreading. It is the result of new conflicts that might be brought upon by the very stress of cancer diagnosis or of invasive and painful therapies.

Dr. Hamer started to give psychotherapy to his patients along with the treatment. He felt that as soon as psychotherapy shows its effect, the patient is out of this shock (Psychosomatic), cancer cells stop multiplying and the dark circles of brain start to disappear instantly. X-rays of the brain now showed a healing edema around the damaged emotional centre as the brain tissue began to repair the affected point. There was once again normal communication between brain and body. A similar healing edema could also be seen around the now inactive cancer tissue. Eventually, the cancer would become encapsulated, discharged or dealt with by the natural action of the body. Diseased tissue would disappear and normal tissue would then again appear.

This way Dr. Hamer proved that unavoidable stress or conflict is the cause of cancer and other diseases. The paragraph below shows different psychosomatic trauma or shock and the corresponding cancer it causes.

Organ affected by Cancer and Type of Stress connection

> **Bone -** Lack of self-worth, inferiority feeling
> **Bladder -** Ugly conflict, dirty tricks
> **Breast, right -** Conflict with husband or partner
> **Breast, left -** Conflict concerning child, home, and mother
> **Cervix -** Severe frustration
> **Colon -** Ugly indigestible conflict
> **Esophagus -** Cannot have it or swallow it
> **Lung -** Fear of dying or suffocation, including fear for someone else
> **Kidneys -** Not wanting to live, water or fluid conflict
> **Liver -** Fear of starvation
> **Testes and Ovaries -** Loss conflict

Breast milk gland - Involving care or disharmony
Breast milk duct - Separation conflict
Intestines - Indigestible chunk of anger
Uterus - Sexual conflict
Gall Bladder - Rivalry conflict
Adrenal cortex - Wrong direction, gone astray
Larynx - Conflict of fear and fright
Bronchials - Territorial conflict
Skin - Loss of integrity
Prostate - Ugly conflict with sexual connections or connotations
Melanoma - feeling dirty, soiled, defiled
Pancreas - Anxiety-anger conflict with family members, inheritance
Spleen - Shock of being physically or emotionally wounded
Rectum - Fear of being useless
Stomach- Indigestible anger, swallowed too much
Thyroid - Feeling powerless
Mouth - Cannot chew or hold it
Lymph glands - Loss of self-worth associated with the location

Dr. Ryke Geerd Hamer – A controversial doctor

A great innovative scientist Ryke Geerd Hamer was born on May 17, 1935 in Meltmann in Germany and grew up in Friesland. At 18, he started a medical and Theology studies in Tübingen University, where he fell in love with a medical student named Sigrid Oldenburg whom he married a year later.

He completed his degree in Theology and completed studies of Medicine in 1962 and he got his medical registration in 1963. In 1972 he received the Doctor of Medicine degree in internal medicine and began treating cancer patients in the Tübingen University clinic. He was very intelligent and he made many inventions, including the non-traumatic Scalpel (which was 20 times sharper than the ordinary razor blade), bone cutting saws for plastic surgery and automated massage tables, etc.

He earned lot of money from these inventions and started a clinic in Rome. On August 18, 1978 early morning, a rampaging Italian Prince Victor Emanuel of Savoy shot his son Dirk, who slept unaware in a boat. He was badly injured. Father took care of his son day and night. But on December 7, 1978 Dirk ultimately died in his arms. This was a big shock for the parents. He suffered a loss conflict and after three years he developed cancer in testes. After few months his wife also developed breast cancer. He thought it was the result of the shock of his son's death. Dr. Hamer later named this type of shock, the "Dirk Hamer Syndrome" or DHS.

He researched on cancer patients for many years and proved that each disease is caused by some mental trauma or shock. He experimented on 40,000 patients and based on these experiences, made the five rules of the New German Medicine. The results caused a furor among the doctors but they were not ready to accept these findings. His research did not see any benefits.

Finally, in 1981, he presented his research at the University of Tübingen for verification. He wanted that his research should be taught in medical schools, so that the patient could be benefited by this research. But the university refused to even review his research.

There was deep conspiracy against Dr. Hamer; he was sued in 1986 by the University and court ordered to confiscate his medical registration. Though his research papers could not be denied in the court. But he did not give up and fought for the truth and science for whole of his life. His wife could not come out of son's death agony and eventually died in 1985.

In 1997, he was accused of examining three patients without charging any fee and sent to jail for 19 months as he had no Medical Registration that time. Police took all his research papers and books when he was arrested. His research, study and treatment was so effective that the Public Prosecutor had to admit in the court that 6500 late-stage cancer patients were treated by him, five years later 6,000 of them were still alive.

September 9, 2004 he was arrested again at his residence in Spain, and sent to prison in France. This time he was accused that some French patients died after they read his book, while he never met and consulted these patients. He was released from prison February, 2006 and in March 2007, he was sent to Sendiyard, Norway. Today he has been living in exile in Norway. This is the price he paid for truly serving the humanity.

Journalists and medical experts portray Dr. Hamer as a quack, a self acclaimed miracle healer, a cult leader, or an insane criminal who denied cancer patients the "life-saving" conventional treatments.

Stages of Cancer Development

Phase 1: Inescapable Shock

Phase 1 starts about 18-24 months prior to cancer diagnosis. This is where the person with cancer experiences an unavoidable and prolonged emotional stress or trauma, affecting deep sleep and the production of melatonin. Melatonin, a hormone produced in the pineal gland of the brain during deep sleep, is essential for inhibiting growth of cancer cell and is the primary hormone which regulates the immune system; particularly production of interleukin-2 which controls white blood cell immune functions and protects against microbial infection. Without enough melatonin cancer cells flourish. Dr Hamer proved that every cancer has a specific psycho-emotional cause and a part of the emotional reflex centre in the brain is damaged due to the prolonged stress. And as each part of the emotional reflex centre in the brain controls and is connected to a particular organ of the body. When the emotional centre in the brain breaks down, the organ it controls gets wrong and incomplete signals, becomes cancerous.

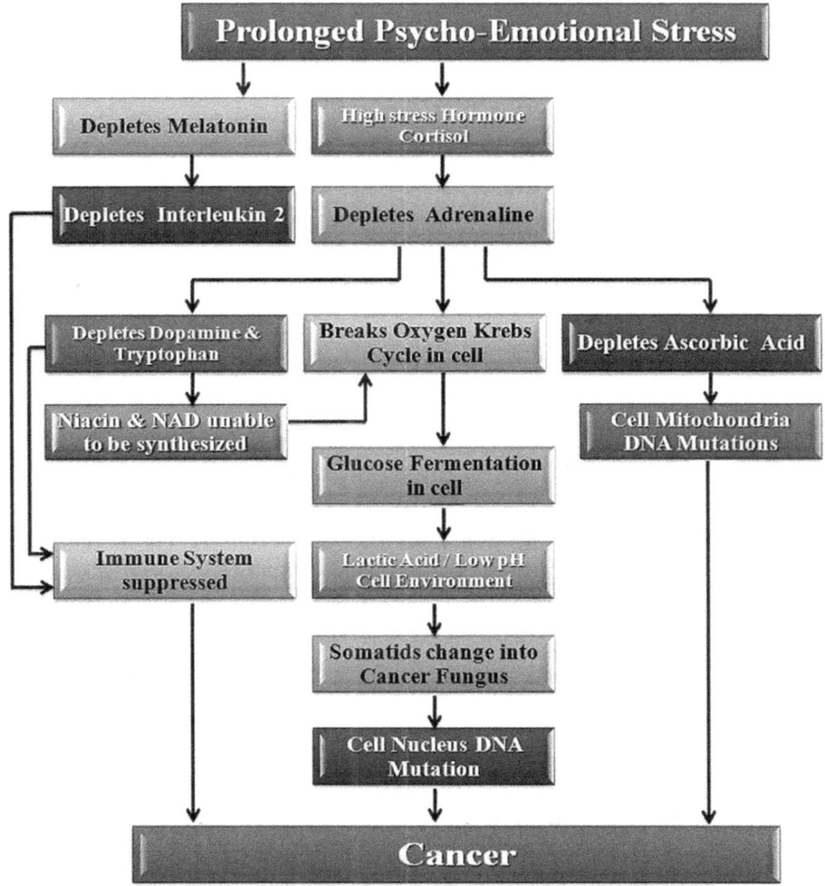

Phase 2: Adrenaline Depletion

In phase 2, stress hormone cortisol levels are raised which deplete adrenaline levels. There are limited reserves of adrenaline in the body and when a person is under constant psycho-emotional stress these reserves are depleted quickly. While insulin helps to shift glucose into cells, the adrenaline is crucial for cell respiration and for converting this glucose into ATP energy for the body and for healthy cell division (which occurs via the metabolic pathway known as Oxidative Phosphorylation and via the Krebs' Citric Acid Cycle in the mitochondria of the cell). Without adrenaline to stimulate production of the GDP molecule (which is essential for mitochondrial cell respiration and glucose conversion), the cells Krebs' Cycle and Oxidative Phosphorylation metabolic pathway is broken and the cell is starts to ferment glucose instead as a means to obtain some amounts of ATP energy (via Glycolysis), which creates lactic acid state in the body and a low pH environment in the cell. This sets the stage for the cancer-fungus to evolve in phase 3 to ferment rising glucose and lactic acid, causing cell mutation.

Phase 3: The Cancer Fungus

In phase 3, somatids (small microorganisms essential for life) that live in our cells pleomorphise into yeast-like-fungus to ferment excess glucose and produce lactic acid in cells (due to the cell fermenting glucose for energy caused by a broken Krebs' Cycle). In a healthy person, somatids have 3 stages in their life cycle – somatid, spore, double spore. However, in a highly acidic low pH lactic acid environment, somatids pleomorphise into a further 13 stages. These stages include viral-bacterial-yeast-like-fungus forms which ferment excess glucose and produce lactic acid in the cell. These fungal pathogenic forms then shift to the cell nucleus to produce waste products called mycotoxins, inhibits repair of cell DNA and also inhibit the very important tumor suppressor genes. Without this gene p53 which regulate cell death (apoptosis), the cell mutation starts beyond repair, and 'cell-growth regulating' proto-oncogenes turn into oncogenes, causing normal cells to mutate into cancer cells.

Phase 4: Niacin Deficiency

In phase 4, depleted adrenaline (epinephrine) levels cause a depletion of dopamine in the brain. Adrenaline is made by dopamine, and as more and more dopamine is used up during stress, the amino-acid tryptophan creates serotonin to please the depressed mood. This causes a depletion of tryptophan which is required to produce niacin/niacinamide (vitamin B3) for cell respiration. Normally tryptophan converts niacin into NAD coenzymes which are then required by the Krebs' Citric Acid Cycle in the mitochondria for cell respiration, glucose conversion and the creation of ATP energy. Without niacin and NAD coenzymes, the Krebs's Citric Acid Cycle is broken, causing the cell to ferment glucose for energy, resulting in cell mutation and the formation of cancer.

Phase 5: Vitamin C Deficiency

In phase 5, depleted adrenaline levels cause a depletion of ascorbic acid (vitamin C) in the adrenal glands. Ascorbic acid is the important substance used by dopamine to make noradrenaline in the adrenal glands, which is then converted to adrenaline. During prolonged stress more and more adrenaline is depleted, meaning more and more ascorbic acid is used up in the creation of adrenaline. During chronic stress the adrenal glands also release ascorbic acid into the body to diminish the stressful impact of adrenaline on the heart and blood pressure. Ascorbic acid is essential for preventing cell DNA damage caused by "oxidative stress", converting oxygen waste products superoxide and hydrogen peroxide into oxygen and water within the cell mitochondria throughout the Oxidative Phosphorylation. The continual loss of ascorbic acid (during prolonged chronic stress) thereby increases DNA damage and mutation in cell mitochondria, causing normal cells to turn into cancer.

Phase 6: Immune Suppression

In phase 6, the immune system becomes weaker by a subconscious desire to "exit life"; due to elevated stress hormone cortisol levels depleting serotonin and dopamine levels in the brain that cause internal depression. An individual experiencing prolonged stress becomes tired of life and wants to come out of the never-ending stress and pain of life, by sending messages to the immune system to shut down. This occurs at the subconscious level where the immune system receives signals to stop production of interleukin-2- producing T cells, B cells, natural killer cells, macrophages and neutrophils. Without immune defenses, viral-bacterial-yeast-like-fungus that have pleomorphised within cells in phase 3 continue to grow and newly produced cancer cells go on multiplying.

How to Heal the Psycho-Emotional Trauma

The diagnosis of cancer is not a death certificate; it just shows you that your physical, emotional, mental and spiritual bodies are out of balance. It is a simple warning to you that you have not healed old wounds. These should be identified and healed. Hammer suggested the following treatments to resolve the Psycho-Emotional conflict:

1. You can consult experienced healer/therapist to heal these wounds. Many CDs and guides are available to help you in heal deeper layers of buried emotions in your subconscious mind.

2. According to Lothar Hirneise, 100% of all late stage 'miracle' cancer survivors had all made considerable **"systems change"** in their lives. This means they had all either left their stressful jobs, ended troubled marriages, shifted to other places or countries for the purpose of removing all stress from their lives.

3. Cancer patients often do not have proper sleep and thus do not produce enough **Melatonin**. Remember that melatonin is also produced during meditation. So meditate for at least 30 minutes a day or take melatonin orally.

4. High stress hormone cortisol levels deplete adrenaline reserves in the body. It is essential to include one daily activity to relax your mind, for the purpose of reducing stress hormone cortisol levels. Optimally spend 2 hours per day in relaxation. This can include walking on the beach, sitting amongst nature, undertaking yoga, yoga nidra or divine sleep, massage, meditation or visualization.

5. High stress hormone cortisol, low melatonin levels, parasites, pathogenic microbes, chemotherapy and

radiation all weaken the immunity. So it is very important to support the immune system during recovery from cancer. We recommend you incorporate at least one therapy to boost and support your immune system. High dose Vitamin C therapy can be used. Visualization helps boost your Immunity. Consider graviola fruit to prevent side-effects of chemotherapy or radiation. Remember that graviola is not compatible with Budwig Diet.

6. Removing the Cancer-Fungus, without which Cancer could not exist. Prolonged psycho-emotional stress suppresses the immune power. When the immunity is suppressed, somatids - change from harmless to pathogenic viral-bacterial-yeast-like-fungus forms. Cancer cannot exist without this viral-bacterial-yeast-like fungus. They travel to the cell nucleus and release "mycotoxins" which causes cell DNA damage and the mutation of normal cells into cancer cells, and ferment the glucose in cancer cells. They provide a natural growth factor for cancer cells to metastasize in the body. It is highly recommended you include at least one of the following to remove the cancer-fungus from your body: Apple Cider Vinegar, Garlic, and Soda bicarb, Essiac Tea or Hyperthermia.

7. Toxins which include "mycotoxins" or acidic waste products caused by the cancer-fungus, poor diet, chemicals, alcohol, tobacco, antibiotics, chemo-therapy, fermentation, poor exercise causing build-up of lactic acid, and dead microbes, parasites and cancer cells. These toxins accumulate in the liver which is the master immune system organ. When the liver is flooded with these toxins, the immune system is weakened and you feel sick, and cancer cells, viral-bacterial-yeast-like-fungus thrives. It is very important to detox the liver, colon (the intestinal immune system), as well as the gall bladder and kidneys, to prevent toxin build up within your body. When you are killing the cancer-fungus or cancer cells using an

alternative or orthodox approach, you should detox the body at the same time, because your liver cannot remove all the dead microbes and cancer cells being killed in the process from the body. We suggest you to include at least one therapy to detox the liver and colon on regular basis e.g. **Liver-Colon Cleanse and Coffee Enema**. Ozonated Water should be strongly considered for it is a super body detoxifier, except lung cancer patients or lung disease.

8. Niacin (Vitamin B3) is a critical element needed by the body's cells to function in a healthy way. Without niacin, the Krebs' Cycle of cells is broken or impaired, and the cell reverts to glycolysis and the fermenting of glucose to obtain energy, causing cancer to develop. **Vitamin C** can be given 12 grams per day without much difficulty. 500 mg to 1500 mg **Niacin** (Tab. Neasyn-SR 500) is prescribed per day.

9. Cancer cells can only survive in low pH or acidic environment caused by the lactic acid produced during fermentation and by viral-bacterial-yeast-like-fungus excreting "mycotoxins" within cells. As cancer cells find it difficult to survive in an alkaline environment of 7.5 or greater, so it is essential to include a 3-step program to restore correct cell pH, which includes: **1) alkaline foods, 2) the removal of lactic-acid forming emotional stress and 3) the dextrorotatory lactic acid which is a key ingredient in sauerkraut and cottage cheese.**

10. Cancer sometimes manifests as a direct result of a subconscious desire to "exit life", caused by the individual feeling overwhelmed by the pains of life and no longer having a strong desire to live. This desire to exit life sends messages to the immune system to shut down. This subconscious desire to exit life must be reversed in order to survive cancer. **Visualization** and guided-imagery tools help to both heal and reverse this subconscious death wish

11. **Prayer** connects you to God and helps to overcome the subconscious death wish. When we asked what is the best option to cure last stage cancer, the first reply is a prayer. Ask God to forgive you for any wrong-doings, Tell Him to fill your life with love, health and happiness and diminish pain.

After I presented a lecture in Vienna in May 1991, a doctor gave me a brain computer tomogram (CT) of a patient. In the presence of 20 of my colleagues, among them radiologists and computer tomography experts, one radiologist asked me to tell him what symptoms the patient had and which type of conflicts where related to them. I was asked to conclude from the brain level the condition of the other two levels. I diagnosed from the brain CT a freshly bleeding bladder carcinoma in the healing phase, an old prostate carcinoma, a diabetic condition, an old bronchial carcinoma, and a sensory paralysis of a certain area in the body and for each of these, the corresponding conflicts that the patient must have experienced. At this point the doctor stood up in front of all his colleagues and said, "Dr. Hamer, congratulations! Five diagnoses - five successes! The patient had exactly what you say. And you were even able to differentiate what symptoms he had in the past and which symptom he has right now."

Dr. Ryke Geerd *Hamer*

Emotional Freedom Technique

Effective Energy Balancing Method That Addresses All Issues

Emotional Freedom Technique is a relatively new discovery and a fast-evolving magical treatment which works by releasing blockages within the energy system and provides rapid relief from physical-emotional issues (e.g. trauma, phobia, grief, anger, Guilt, anxiety, nightmares, depression, pain, headaches and much more). This is based on 5000 year old energy healing techniques such as acupuncture or qigong. This energy, which flows in energy meridians, is called "chi" or "qi" in China.

This Technique is also called Emotional Acupuncture, which involves the use of fingertips rather than needles to tap on the end points of energy meridians that are situated just beneath the surface of the skin.

When your computer hangs or overburdens, you simply press the "Restart Button", then it restarts and start working normally. EFT works just like a "Restart Button" of the body's energy system.

The main goal of this article is to teach you with an easy to use recipe to achieve emotional freedom. You can call it EFT or Emotional Freedom Technique. Now you are going to learn how to do basic steps of EFT in detail. You will use this recipe in every session, whether you are a beginner or experienced.

Although I am going to describe EFT procedure in detail, But the Basic Recipe (how to do EFT) has only 5 brief steps (ingredients) and you can learn easily. Once you have learned the recipe, you can perform a single round in about 30 seconds. It may require some practice, of course, but after a few tries the whole process becomes very easy and you can do it even in your sleep. You will then have a wonderful tool which you can use for a lifetime.

We apply The Basic Recipe to every emotional, physical and performance issue. It doesn't matter whether the problem is big or small, complicated or impossible it may look; we still use the same Basic Recipe. We may aim the process in sophisticated ways but the tapping process remains the same.

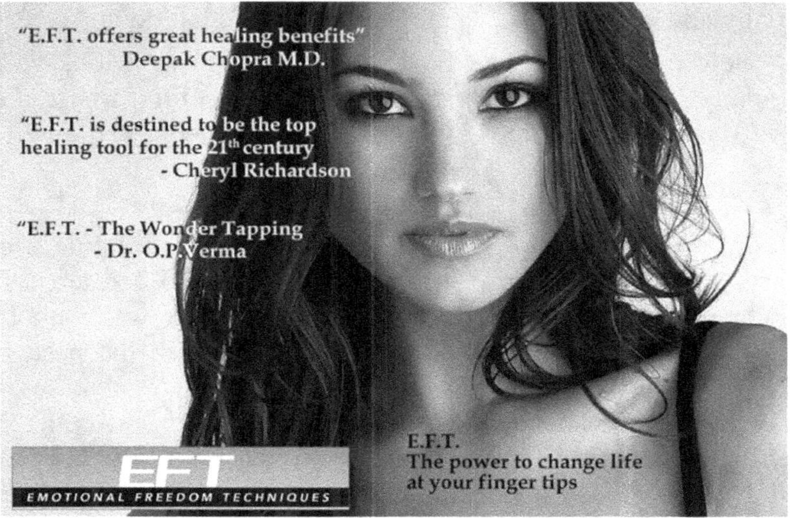

EFT is an effective way to balance the energy system to address all issues that have emotional causes. Grief, anger, guilt, depression, trauma, fear etc. are simple Emotional issues. And since both physical and performance issues are often caused by emotional issues, that's why one energy balancing technique e.g. EFT can be useful for all of them.

The Basic Recipe blends simple verbal commands with a 9 point tapping sequence. The verbal commands tell our system what we working on and what we want our energy system to do. These commands are an essential part of the process. The tapping at specific points stimulates the energy pathways and tells them to balance the energy disruptions. These points we use are at or near the end points of the energy pathways (meridians and vessels). In acupuncture over 300 meridian points are used while just a few are used by EFT. EFT represents a different use of these pathways and allows someone with no formal training in Chinese medicine to get wonderful results with a simple process.

In practice, the 14 energy pathways in the body are interconnected and so sending balancing command to one pathway affects other pathways. This is the reason why we usually address only a few pathways to get the job done.

Before you learn The Basic Recipe, (1) have a look at the Tapping Points, (2) set the stage with some useful Tapping Tips and (3) review the 5 Steps in The Basic Recipe.

History

In 1980 Psychiatrist Dr. Roger Callahan was treating a girl Mary, a patient of intense water phobia. She also had terrifying nightmares and sharp headache, related with her water phobia. Mary had been treated by several psychiatrists in the past, but could not recover from her illness. Callahan treated her by conventional means for a year and half, but without any significant benefit. During that period Roger was studying body's energy system. Hence he thought to step out of the way and decided to tap with his fingers under her eye (an end point of the stomach meridian).

As soon as he tapped below her eye, she shouted loudly and complained of some stomach discomfort. Surprisingly she immediately told that her phobia was gone. She ran to a nearby swimming pool and began throwing water on her face and body. She was instantly relieved of fear, headache and nightmares. She was totally free of her water phobia. Callahan continued this research and proved that **"The cause of all negative emotions is a disruption in the body's energy system."** This is also called The Discovery Sentence of EFT (Craig, March 15, 2011).

He then integrated acupuncture and kinesiology to develop thought field therapy. He taught this to Gary Crag, a Stanford trained engineer. Gary refined this technique through trial and error and finally developed this wonder art of tapping for removing the negative emotions. He called this Emotional Freedom Technique.

The Tapping Points

Try to locate each of the points on your body and touch each of them with your fingers.

- **The Karate Chop point KC:** The Karate Chop point (often called KC) is located at the center of the fleshy part of the inner side of your hand (both hands) between the top of the wrist and the base of the little finger or simply the part of your hand you use to give a karate chop.
- **Top of Head Point TOH:** On the top of the head. If you were to draw a line from one ear, over the head, to the other ear, and another line from your nose to the back of your necks center, the TOH point is where these two lines intercept.
- **Eye Brow Point EB:** At the beginning of the eyebrow, just above and to one side of the nose. This is often called EB for the Eye Brow point.
- **Side of the Eye Point SE:** On the bone bordering the outside corner of the eye. This is often called SE for Side of the Eye point.
- **Under the Eye Point UE:** On the bone under an eye about 1 inch below your pupil. This is often called UE for Under the Eye point.
- **Under Nose Point UN:** On the small area between the bottom of your nose and the top of your upper lip. This is often called UN for Under the Nose point.
- **Chin Point Ch:** Midway between the point of your chin and the bottom of your lower lip. Though it is not directly on the point of the chin, it is called chin point, very near to chin. This is often called Ch for Chin point.
- **Collar Bone Point CB:** The junction where the sternum (breastbone), collarbone and the first rib meet. To locate it, first place your index finger on the U-shaped notch at the top of the breastbone. From the bottom of the U shape

notch in your lower neck, move your index finger down toward the navel 1 inch and then go to 1 inch laterally. This point is often called CB for Collar Bone point even though it is not on the collarbone (or clavicle). It is at the beginning of the collarbone and easier to call it the collarbone point.

- **Under Arm Point UA:** On the side of the body below axilla, at a level of the nipple (for men) or in the middle of the bra strap (for women). It is about 4 inches below the armpit. This is often called UA for Under the Arm point.

Tapping Tips

These tips may answer your common questions.

- Some tapping points have twin points on each side of the body.
- For "eyebrow" point on the right side of the body has a twin point on the left side too. Though you only need to tap one of these twin points. But if you have both hands free you can certainly tap on both sides for better approach.
- You can also switch sides when you tap these twin points. For example, during the same round of The Basic Recipe, you can tap the "karate chop" point on your left hand and the eyebrow point on the right side of your body. This makes the tapping process easier to perform.
- The tapping is usually done with two or more fingertips. So that you can cover a larger area and hence insure that you are tapping over the correct point.
- While you can tap with the fingertips of either hand, most people use their dominant hand. For example, right handed people tap with the fingertips of their right hand while left handed people tap with the fingertips of their left hand.
- You should tap approximately 5 times on each point, but there is no need to count the taps because anywhere between 3 and 7 taps is okay. The only exception is during the Setup step, where the Karate Chop Point is

tapped continuously while you repeat some standard wording.

- The process is easy to memorize. After you have tapped the Karate Chop Point, the rest of the points go down the body. The Eyebrow point, for example, is below the Top of the Head point. The Side of the Eye point is below the Eyebrow point. And so on down the body.

The 5 Steps of the Basic Recipe

EFT process can be memorized easily.

1. Identify the issue: Here you make a mental picture of your issue in simple and clear words. This becomes the target at which you focus the Basic Recipe. Examples might be: **a severe headache or fear of spiders.** Remember you should only target one issue at a time. As you will learn later, trying to combine issues in the process will compromise your results.

2. Test the Initial Intensity of your issue: The basic scale we use for testing the intensity was developed by a famous psychiatrist called Joseph Wolpe in the 1950s and called Subjective Units of Disorder (SUD), because you measure the intensity by your judgment. This measures our degree of discomfort on a scale of 0 to 10. Zero indicates no discomfort, and 10 is the maximum possible distress. This scale works equally well for psychological problems such as anxiety and physical problems such as pain. This serves as a reference so that we can compare our progress after each round of The Basic Recipe. If, for example, we started at an 8 and eventually reach at 4, then we know we have achieved a 50% improvement. The number of possible issues we can address with The Basic Recipe is endless.

3. The Setup: The Setup is a process we use to start each round of tapping. By designing a simple phrase and saying it while continuously tapping the KC point, you let your system know what you're trying to address. When designing this phrase there are two goals to achieve:

Identify the problem - This involves remembering the problem. You expose your mind repeatedly to the memory of the issue. This is the opposite of what we normally do; we usually want an emotional trauma to fade away. We might engage in behaviors like avoidance so that we don't have to deal with unpleasant memories.

Accept yourself in spite of it - You don't tell yourself that things will get better, or that you'll improve. You simply express the intention of accepting yourself just the way you are. You accept the reality. We do this by saying:

"Even though I have *(name of the problem)*, I deeply and completely accept myself, I love myself." *(name of the problem)* is the problem you want to address, so you can just insert things like: severe headache or fear of spiders.

"Even though I have *severe headache*, I deeply and completely accept myself, I love myself.

Or "Even though I have *fear of spiders*, I deeply and completely accept myself, I love myself."

We do not want to use EFT on someone else's problem. For example, rather than, "Even though my son is addicted to drugs, I deeply and completely accept myself, I love myself." it's better to focus on your own reaction which might be, "Even though I'm frustrated by my son's drug addiction." We want to aim EFT at our part of the problem rather than trying to fix someone else's problem.

Important, Important, Important: The language that we use always aims at the negative. This is essential because it is the negative that creates the energy disruptions that The Basic Recipe clears (and thus brings peace to the system). By contrast, conventional methods and popular self-help books stress positive thinking and teach to avoid the negative. But in EFT, on the other hand, needs to aim at the negative so it can be neutralized. This allows our energy system to bubble up natural positives to the top.

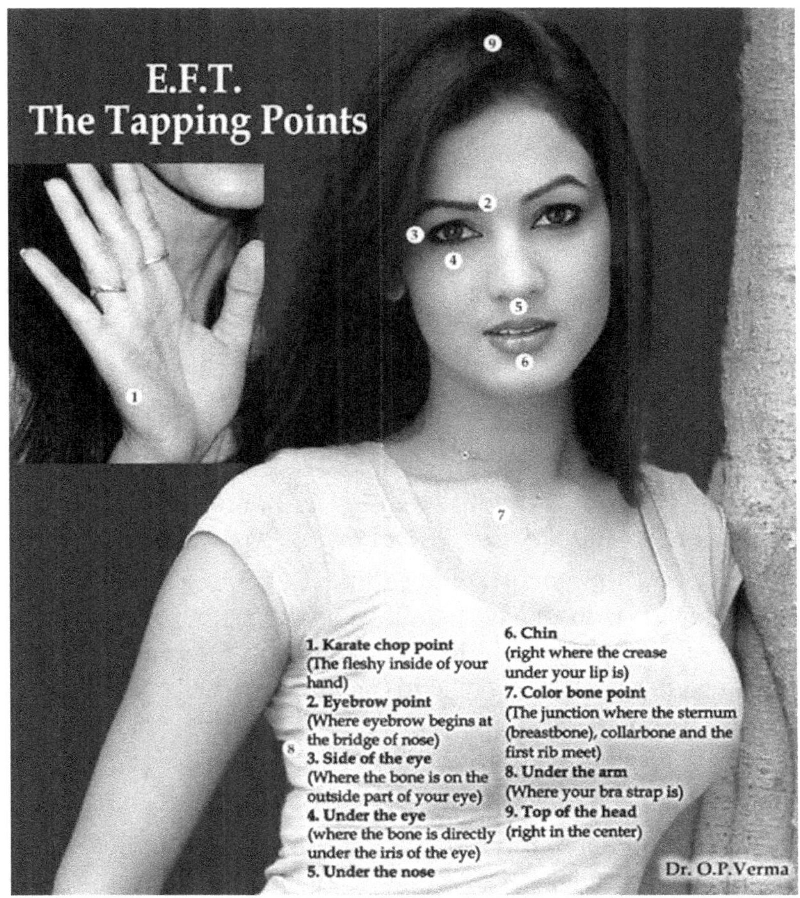

4. The Sequence: This is the workhorse part of The Basic Recipe that stimulates/balances the body's energy pathways. It is the main part of the how to do EFT basics process. Do it 5-7 times. To perform it, you tap each of the tapping points while saying a Reminder Phrase that keeps your system connected into the issue. I list the points below, followed by a description of the Reminder Phrase:

Top of the Head (TOH) Beginning of the Eyebrow (EB) Side of the Eye (SE) Under the Eye (UE) Under the Nose (UN) Chin

131

Point (CH) Beginning of the Collarbone (CB) Under the Arm (UA)

The Reminder Phrase is quite simple as you need only acknowledge the issue with some brief wording. Depending on your issue, you might say the following at each tapping point.... *"This headache", or "this fear of spiders."*

5. Test the Intensity Again and Repeat if necessary: Finally, you again measure the level of issue's intensity by assigning a number to it on a 0-10 scale. You compare this with the initial level to see how much progress you have made. If you are not down to zero then repeat the process until you either achieve zero or as low as possible. When you repeat the sequence, you should add the word **"Remaining"** before the Reminder Phrase. So your Reminder Phrase should be...... *"Remaining headache", or "Remaining fear of spiders."*

You can also include some additional tapping points that will be introduced in the next section. Now I assume that you have familiarized yourself with the Tapping Points, Tapping Tips and the 5 Steps to the Basic Recipe given above.

6. Now take a deep breath.

The 9 Gamut Procedure

This is, perhaps, the most bizarre procedure in EFT. It was originally designed by Dr. Roger Callahan. It "fine tunes" the brain via some tapping sequence along with eye movements, some humming and counting. Certain parts of the brain are stimulated through connecting nerves, when the eyes are moved. Likewise the right side of the brain (the creative side) is engaged when you hum a song and the left side (the digital side) is engaged when you count. Therapists rarely use this procedure these days. It is helpful when there is a clear brain disorder (e.g. Cerebral Palsy) and once in a while if The Basic Recipe doesn't work. It will occasionally make a difference.

The 9 Gamut Procedure is a short procedure in which a set of 9 "brain stimulating" actions are performed while continuously tapping on the Gamut Point. To do the 9 Gamut Procedure, you must first locate the Gamut point. It is on the back of either hand, about 1/2 inch above the midpoint between the knuckles at the base of the ring finger and the little finger.

Next, you must perform 9 different actions while tapping the Gamut point continuously. The 9 Gamut actions are:

1. Eyes closed.

2. Eyes open.

3. Eyes looking down right while holding the head steady.

4. Eyes looking down left while holding the head steady.

5. Roll your eyes in a circle clockwise as if your nose is at the center of a clock and you were trying to see all the numbers in order.

6. Roll your eyes in a circle anti-clockwise as if your nose is at the center of a clock and you were trying to see all the numbers in reverse order.

7. Hum a song again for 2 seconds (any song of your choice).

8. Count 1 to 5 numbers rapidly.

9. Hum a song again for 2 seconds.

Note that these 9 actions are presented in a certain order and I suggest that you memorize them in the given order. However, you can mix the order up if you wish so long as you do all 9 of them.... and.... you perform 7, 8 & 9 as a unit. That is, you hum 2 seconds of a song (can hum Happy Birthday to you) ... then count ... then hum the song again, in that order. However, you could also change the order of 7, 8 & 9 from hum-count-hum to count-hum- count. Either option will suffice.

Living with Cancer and EFT

Cancer is a troublesome path of life, full of pain and sorrows that one doesn't choose to take. Though EFT does NOT claim a cure for cancer, but is a powerful modality for managing the associated emotional trauma, helping to calm and rebalance the energy system and clear the blocks in the healing process, both physical and emotional. The beauty of EFT is that it can be used with any treatment. During journey of treating cancer one can feel very weak and helpless due to many factors such as with the side effects of chemotherapy, radiotherapy etc. and with the trauma associated with surgery. EFT gives a new hope of getting some control and actively helping in healing process.

Often cancer diagnosis causes stress and emotional trauma. Use EFT to clear the trauma of diagnosis from energy system. The connection between trauma or shock and cancer is well documented and re-searched, so this initial treatment to clear the physiological impact of the diagnosis is vitally important.

The first thing that needs to focus after diagnosis is decision of selecting a right treatment, often done in extreme urgency, stress and anxiety. EFT allows clearing the confusion and taking a right decision. Here you need not focus on any specific set-up statement or reminder phrase, just tap continually on the points to rebalance and restore your system.

The word 'cancer' too can create fear. It can be extremely useful to begin a few rounds EFT of simply repeating the word 'cancer' until the fear reduces and word cancer becomes just like any other word. This does not mean you will feel indifferent to it, but that it loses its negative impact on your system and clears up your energy to focus on healing.

Often a cancer diagnosis brings some lifestyle changes immediately such as giving up smoking, drugs, alcohol, change in nutrition or financial implications. EFT is a very good tool that can help to this change over.

EFT provides an effective way of managing ones emotional state and reducing any pain, fears and anxiety. However, it is also very important to resolve underlying core issues which may be contributing to the creation of the cancer, negative emotions and traumas that still block our energy system. (Craig, March 15, 2011)

Coconut Oil - The Unique Designer Fat

To date, there are over 1,500 studies proving coconut oil (Cocos nucifera) to be one of the healthiest oil on the planet. Coconut oil benefits and uses go beyond what most people realize. Coconut has long been a primary source of food throughout the tropics. Its various industrial and cosmetic applications have made it a very important commodity. Coconut oil is heat stable, resists rancidity and has a shelf life of approximately two years or more. The best coconut oil is raw, unrefined, unheated, cold-pressed, "extra virgin" and organic.

World's renowned expert of fats and oils and the chief expert at the Federal Institute for Fats Research, Germany, and Dr Johanna Budwig scientifically proved that good quality coconut oil is the best oil for high temperature cooking, e.g. frying and deep frying. **It does not change into Tran's fatty acids when heated.** She recommended only Coconut oil for cooking to her Cancer patients.

Composition

The coconut possesses a wide variety of health benefits due to its fiber and nutritional content, but it is the oil that makes it a remarkable source of food and medicine. It has definitely earned its reputation as the healthiest oil in the world despite the fact that its high saturated fat content was once falsely claimed to be unhealthy.

Coconut oil - The best source of The MCFAs

Oils and fats are composed of molecules known as fatty acids. They are classified either according to saturation or based on molecular length and size of the carbon chain within each fatty acid. Monounsaturated fats and polyunsaturated fats are an example of the first class.

The second classification is based on molecular size or length of the fatty acids carbon chain. Long chains of carbon atoms consist of each fatty acid with an attached hydrogen atom. There are short chain fatty acids known as SCFA, medium chain fatty acids (MCFA) such as coconut oil and long chain fatty acids (LCFA). The majority of fats and oils in our diet (whether unsaturated or saturated) are composed of long chain fatty acids.

Coconut oil is predominantly medium-chain fatty acid (MCFA) and the effects of the MCFA in coconut oil are distinctly different from the LCFA found in other foods. Why is this relevant? It is important because our bodies respond and metabolize each fatty acid differently. It is the MCFA found in coconut oil that makes it unique because these fatty acids do not have a negative effect on cholesterol. In fact, they are known to lower the risk of heart disease and atherosclerosis. There are only few dietary sources of MCFA, and one of the best sources is coconut oil.

But the people who are blind followers of FDA and AHA (American Heart Association) will never believe these facts because they have very narrow and tubular vision where saturation is the only criteria to judge the fats.

Medium-chain fats leave the stomach altogether unaltered and do not need any fat-splitting enzymes or gallic acid for their digestion. These designer and unique fatty acids are small and tender enough to slip easily into mitochondria – the cells' powerhouses – directly where they can then be converted to energy. Therefore, it is not true that these fats would contribute to arterial calcification. Another reason for the use of coconut fat is the fact that it helps to absorb other substances such as magnesium, calcium, certain B vitamins, fat-soluble vitamins (A, D, E and K) and even certain proteins. Around 62% of the oils in coconut are made up of these 3 healthy fatty acids and 91% of the fat in coconut oil is healthy saturated fat. **These unique fats include:**

- **Lauric acid**

- **Caprylic acid**
- **Capric acid**

Coconut oil has many health benefits which are attributed to the presence of lauric acid. Lauric acid is converted into a monoglyceride called monolaurin, a compound that is highly toxic to viruses, bacteria, fungus and other microorganisms because of its ability to disrupt their lipid membranes and virtually destroy them. Monolaurin is effective for treating candida albicans, fungal infections and athlete's foot.

In natural medicine, coconut fat plays an important role in the treatment of inflammation, bacterial and viral infections and even fungi. The well-known AIDS study conducted by Philippine San Lazaro Hospital showed that coconut fat is able to reduce the viral load and causes the CD4 to increase in AIDS patients. It also has positive effects in such known viruses as influenza, herpes simplex or the Epstein-Barr virus.

Breast milk is the only other source of lauric acid, which must explain the lesser incidents of infections with breast-fed infants. It has also been observed that regular consumption of coconut oil boosts immunity and reduces incidences of sickness.

Health benefits

Hair Care - The unique MCFAs in coconut oil pass freely into the hair's cell membrane, allowing for the oil to penetrate the hair's shaft; this literally does the deep conditioning from within.

Massaging the oil into the scalp can offer relief from dandruff. Dandruff is caused by dry skin or fungal condition that reached the scalp. With regular use, coconut oil can kill the fungus and eliminate dandruff issues.

Skin Care - Coconut oil is an excellent skin conditioner containing MCFAs, naturally occurring fats which deeply penetrate, moisturize and acts as a protective barrier against environmental and free radical damage. The oil also provides sun protection by screening 20 percent of ultraviolet exposure.

Coconut oil is rich in anti-oxidants and the natural antibacterial agents caphrylic and capric acids. Its ability to smooth the skin while infusing with anti-oxidants makes it a perfect anti-aging moisturizer. Moreover, it contains vitamin E, another antioxidant popular for hastening the recovery of skin abrasions, burns and other trauma.

Weight Loss - Medium-chain fatty acids found in coconut oil can speed up metabolism three times faster than long-chain fatty acids because they are easily digested and converted into energy.

Hypothyroidism – Coconut oil has been found to be very helpful for people who have hypothyroidism. It has been scientifically proved to increase metabolism, encourages weight loss, increases body temperature, relieves constipation and behaves as an antioxidant. Thyroid patients often experience muscle and joint pain due to inflammation from unbalanced hormone levels. Coconut oil naturally suppresses inflammation and helps to repair tissues and fight pain.

Low thyroid hormones in the body can cause dry skin. coconut oil helps to restore the lost moisture and improve skin health. A thyroid disorder can also affect the hair follicles. Lauric acid provides the protein required by hair to stay healthy and strong, to reduce hair loss. Use extra virgin and organic Coconut oil. The amount varies between 3 to 6 tablespoons a day.

It should be noted that ninety-three percent of American soy is GMO. This highly processed soy has been linked to **thyroid damage and hormone disruption** due to its large quantities of estrogen-like compounds called phytoestrogens.

Natural remedy for Pneumonia - In a study presented before The American College of Chest Physicians on October 29, 2008, coconut oil was found to offer pneumonia patients faster and more complete relief from symptoms.

Diabetes, Heart Disease and Cholesterol levels - In a study made on women subjects ranging from 20 to 40 years old, half of the subjects were instructed to take a 30 ml soybean oil supplement while the other half were instructed to take a 30 ml coconut oil supplement while maintaining moderate exercise routine over a 12 week period. Results of the study showed that although both group of women had a decrease in body mass index (BMI), only the women who were taking coconut oil showed a notable decease in waist circumference significantly lowering the risk of conditions like type II diabetes and heart disease.

Furthermore, the study also showed that the subjects who experienced an improvement in their cholesterol profile along with higher HDL levels and higher HDL/LDL ratio were the ones taking coconut oil. That taking soybean oil did not receive the same benefits but reflected higher total cholesterol as well as higher LDL cholesterol, lower HDL cholesterol and a lower HDL/LDL ratio.

Bone health and Chronic fatigue - Coconut oil help prevent osteoporosis because it helps in the nutrient absorption of minerals such as calcium and magnesium - important minerals that fight osteoporosis. Moreover, the MCFAs in coconut oil produce energy rather than body fat, thereby improving metabolism and preventing fatigue.

Alzheimer's Disease - Dr. Mary Newport gave her husband 1 Tbsp. of coconut oil twice a day for a month and a half and saw him almost completely recovered from dementia.

Plethora of others health benefits
- Protects against cancer, HIV and other infectious diseases
- Kills bacteria and parasites like tape worm and liver flukes
- Eases acid reflux, aids in proper bowel function
- Lowers incidence of hemorrhoids
- Heals and relieves intestinal problems
- Soothes earaches
- Deals with symptoms connected with prostate enlargement
- Strengthens the liver and protects against degeneration

- Reduces incidence of epileptic seizures
- Reduces joint and muscle inflammation
- Eases neuropathies and itching from diabetes.

Dose of Coconut Oil to enjoy its benefits

There is no real dose of recommended coconut oil, but research has shown that one should consume several grams of lauric acid, or at least **1 Tbsp of coconut oil, every day**. Certainly 10 g to 20 g of lauric acid taken daily can be a benefit to health. Coconut oil contains 50 percent lauric acid, so taking 1 tablespoon of coconut oil per day will provide you with 7g lauric acid. An appropriate dose should therefore be in the region of one to three tablespoons daily.

Testimonials

How Dr. Siegfried Ernst cured his stomach cancer

Great healing story written by Dr. Robert Willner

Biography of Dr. Robert Willner

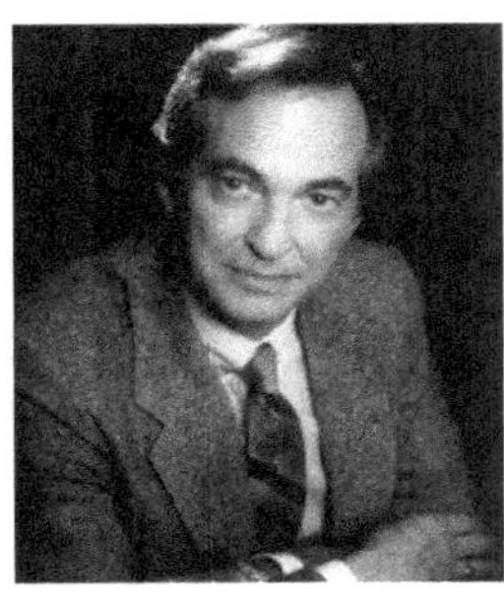

Dr. Robert Willner M.D., PhD (21 June 1929 - 15 April 1995) was an American doctor remembered for his role in AIDS denialism, the view that AIDS is not caused by HIV infection. Willner described himself as originally an "orthodox" physician who slowly changed to alternative medicine, particularly after his wife died of cancer chemotherapy.

In 1995, Willner stated that "I am fully convinced; you can prevent all disease with diet, lifestyle changes and sanitation." Willner wrote some books presenting his point of view on the relation between HIV and AIDS, titled "Deadly Deception: the Proof That Sex And HIV Absolutely Do Not Cause AIDS". The book was published shortly after Wilmer's medical license was revoked for, among other things, treating an AIDS patient with ozone therapy. He also wrote a book about cancer "The Cancer Solutions" after he met Dr. Budwig and studied her protocol in detail.

The following month, on October 28, 1994, in a press conference at a Greensboro, North Carolina hotel, Willner jabbed his finger with blood he said was from an HIV-infected patient. Willner died on April 15, 1995 of heart attack.

Lunch with Dr. Siegfried Ernst

Dr. Robert Willner was very much fascinated by Dr. Johanna Budwig and her cancer research. Dr. Budwig presented clear and scientific evidence, which has been confirmed by hundreds of other related research papers since, that the essential fatty acids were at the core of the answer to the cancer problem. He felt compelled to visit Dr. Budwig in Germany and meet her personally so that he would have the very latest information for his book. So he went to Germany several times before completing his book "The Cancer Solutions."

One day at Dr. Johanna Budwig's residence in Freudenstadt, the phone rang and a happy and lively conversation in German ensued. In a few minutes Dr. Budwig asked him to come to take the phone and said. "This is Dr. Ernst, the friend I told you before. Speak with him and confirm anything you would like."

The conversation with Dr, Ernst lasted approximately ten minutes and Willner tried to remember as much as possible. Most of the facts had already been told to him by Dr. Budwig. Then he returned to the hotel, noted down whatever he could recollect. The next day was Friday and he planned to leave in the morning for Stuttgart. His return flight was on Sunday at eight in the morning. Because it required a very early wake-up and he did not want to any risk. So he decided to arrive there a day early. After purchasing as many of Dr. Budwig's books as possible at a local book shop, he took a taxi to the railway station.

The plane that he had hoped to take was full, and he was advised to get a flight from Munich. On the way to Munich the train stopped at Ulm, which in phone conversation, Dr. Ernst had mentioned was his home. He decided to get off the train and try to meet him. Within an hour he had a room in Golden Tulip Hotel and arranged to meet with Dr. Ernst the next morning. That day there was a lot of fog and snow fall in Ulm and weather was scorching cold. He decided to take sauna bath in health club of the hotel. After sauna bath, he felt warm and fresh. He ordered pucked pride dry wine, avocado vasabi salad and hot sizzling fajita for the dinner.

He spent the next day with Dr. Ernst who seemed very healthy and active, though he was in late seventies. He was famous and dedicated man in the town. He was devoted to family, church, city and humanity. The present Pope and many other dignitaries were his close friends.

Dr. Ernst told that seventeen years ago he developed stomach cancer for which he had major surgery. It had required removal of his stomach and left him with a great number of digestive problems and considerable debilitation. His professional life had practically come to an end. He was approximately sixty years old at the time. He had great difficulty in continuing his clinical practice.

Two years later he had a recurrence of the cancer and was advised chemotherapy as the only available remedy. There was very little hope for survival, and he knew that chemotherapy was not only ineffective, but completely damaging for the quality of life, so he said No to chemotherapy.

Then he went to Dr. Budwig for trying her protocol. For two years he religiously followed the Budwig diet and, also, he used the application of the Flax seed oil to his body every evening. The oil was applied to the abdominal area and wrapped with cloth bandages. He continued the low fat Quark and Flax seed oil daily. It has been fifteen years since the recurrence of the stomach cancer and the institution of the Budwig therapy. Dr. Ernst has had healthy life except some minor problems with eating and digesting food. The simple addition of digestive enzymes and other supplements have made his existence almost completely normal.

Virtually all patients with a recurrence of this type of cancer rarely survive a year, even if they agree to chemotherapy. And the toxic-effects from the chemotherapy makes life more regrettable. Of course the conventional doctors will dismiss the story of Dr. Ernst as a "spontaneous remission" in spite of the fact that it is unheard of, except when patients go for simple alternative therapies.

Their conversation lasted for many hours and he confirmed much of what Dr. Budwig had told him. He recalled the many stories of patients she had treated. He admitted that whatever skepticism he had about this great therapy, disappeared completely after meeting with Dr. Ernst. He was both a colleague and a fellow cancer victim who had been truly cured, not just a five-year survival (Dr Robert E. Willner M.D., 1993, Chapter 5).

Highly positive and encouraging story of Mary

Diagnosis of Cancer and the triple bladed sword: surgery, chemo and radio

I was diagnosed with breast cancer in July 2001. I had two surgeries, 47 sessions of radiation and 4 months of chemo.

Then in June 2005, I was told that the cancer had spread to my spine. I underwent a very extensive surgery on June 11, 2005. The doctor told me that cancer was eating my spine and making it weak and hollow. **They said I have 20 months to live.** They explained me that when cancer spreads to your spine; after a few months for it to spread to other organs such as kidneys, bladder, lungs, etc. Then you die. **But first, they wanted give me radiation and chemo again and again until I die.** So in July 2005, I had only 10 sessions of radiation. After this I was totally exhausted and drained. Then I finally decided NO RADIO! NO CHEMO! Nothing! If I am ready to die, I want to enjoy my death!

Starting on my path to healing

No No No ... how could I die so soon! **I would win this war against breast cancer.** So I jumped into the river Google and came out with bunch of research done by a doctor from Germany in my hand. She had developed a simple cure for cancer. Take cold-pressed organic Flax seed oil with Cottage Cheeseand eat only fresh foods, such as veggies and fruits, and get sunlight.

Terminal breast cancer cured in record time

So I had been taking this natural treatment for 8 months? I had my repeat bone scan, MRI and CT in November. **Not only my cancer vanished, but there is new bone growing in the holes where the cancer ate it away!!!** My oncologist is shocked to see the scans! I am thrilled ☺

Winning my cancer war with a bonus:

This time not only have I won the war against cancer, and let's face it... chemo does not CURE cancer. Flax seed oil combined with sulfurated protein is the ONLY CURE for cancer in my experience. I had a scar tissue in my right breast was about the size of a golf ball, shown up on all my mammograms since my surgery in 2001. It was also there in March 2005 as usual. But in the November mammogram, the scar tissue had reduced to the size of a small coin! I fully expect it to be vanished by the mammogram in March 2006! And apart from this healing, I have lost 70 lbs weight! Just from eating right and exercising! Wow! And I look forward to lose another 10 pounds in July. ☺

Breast Cancer - Miracle healing

Mrs. Neelam 60 yrs. from Almoda suffers from Breast Cancer. She came to me in last Dec. She has not taken any Chemo, Radio or Surgery. I advised her to take Budwig Protocol sincerely. She immediately started the Protocol along with Pranayam, Coffee Enema, Soda bicarb bath and Flax oil massage. She called me yesterday on May 1 and told that her tumor has shrieked more than 50%. This is really a miracle of Budwig Protocol.

Wellness Journey of Mrs. Shanti

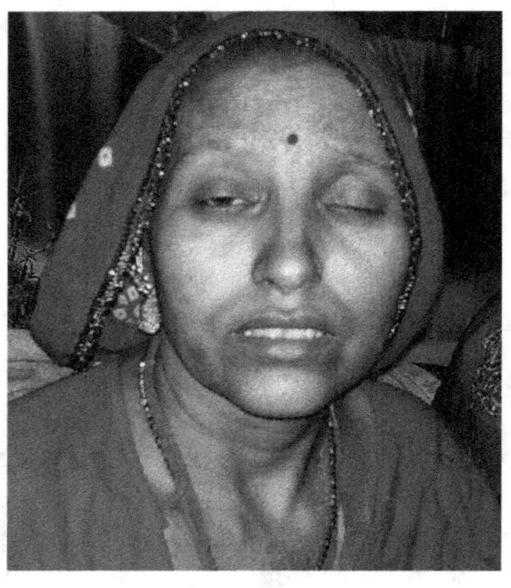

This patient Mrs. Shanti 40 years in age belongs to a village near Dungargarh. She came to us in August, 2014 for the first time. She suffered from Leomyosarcoma Uterus (Cancer of Uterus) before one and half years. She was operated and treated by conventional treatment at Bikaner. She remained in remission for six months. After that she developed Metastasis Tumor in Left Lumbar region. She also had severe anemia (Hb was 5.7 gm in June, 2014), pain, weakness, ascites, anorexia and vomiting. No treatment was helping her. Then somebody told her to consult me. When I examined her she looked very weak, pale, apathic and drowsy, she hardly spoke anything. Her Hemoglobin was approx. 7 Gm. She had unbearable pain in her left Lumbar region.

The whole family was uneducated and lived in farm in rural area. They do not understand Hindi. It was really very difficult for us to train them, as communication was a big problem. But our audio-visual approach helped and conducted the training anyhow. I was very sure that they will hardly follow Budwig Protocol more than a few days. But after a month and half her brother spoke to me and told that patient is improving slowly and asked some questions. It was a bit strange for me but still I had no hope.

On November 25, 2014 when she stepped in to my clinic, I was totally shocked to see her. What a change! What a miracle!! She was entirely a new woman. She looked active, healthy, happy and young. She was smiling, her face was glowing. Her vomiting stopped, appetite improved and pain reduced. She was talking and asking questions in her local language. She followed the Budwig treatment nicely, and she has not taken any conventional treatment during last four months. This time her Hemoglobin was 11.5 Gm, though we did not prescribe her any iron capsule. Her Metastatic tumor which was 84x78x55 mm in June 10, 2014 has reduced to 46x34 mm, a drastic reduction in size. Liver size became normal and kidney stone passed out. This is a magic of Budwig Protocol. This wellness was achieved by use of Flax oil, the sun shine in a bottle or rather the essence of our life.

Many people think that Budwig Protocol is just a mixture of Flax oil and cottage cheese. It is biggest mistake one can ever do. Because in real terms Budwig Protocol is much more than that. It is healing of body, mind and spirit. Here the difference between winning and losing is so small that your minute neglect can tip the balance of the whole treatment. And that is why thorough and 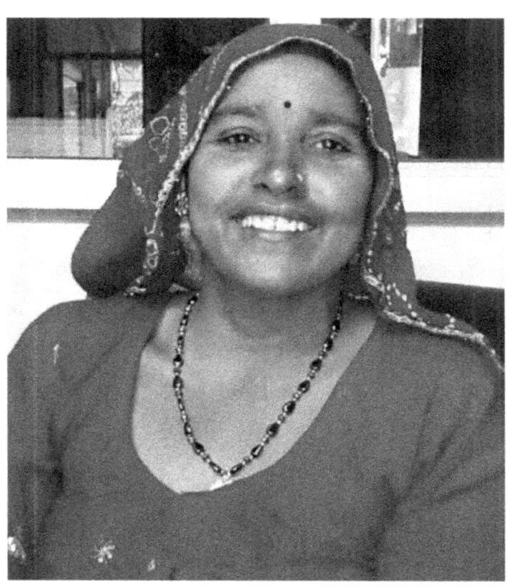 expert training is so important for every patient who wishes to take Budwig Protocol.

Tom's cured his Brain Cancer

My name is Kelly and on February 10, 2002 I brought my husband to the Emergency with a splitting headache and severe vomiting. We thought it was a migraine attack but later found out that it was a brain tumor. On February 12, he had surgery and the biopsy was done. After lab workup surgeon finally declared that he suffered from Glioblastoma Multiforme Grade 4.

The surgeon called me in his office and told me that he removed the tumor as much as he could and Tom had about 6 months to live if he didn't take

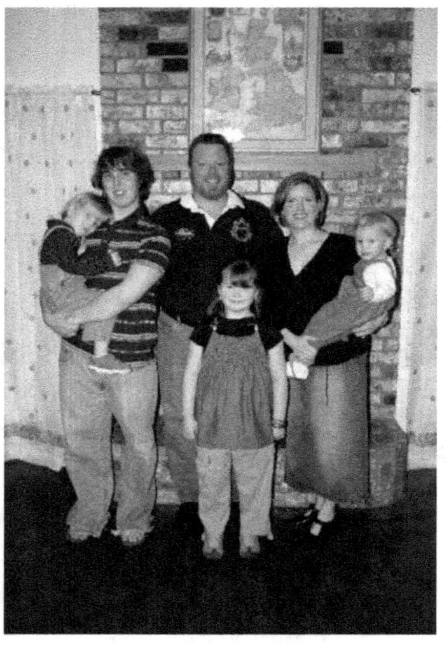

radiotherapy. If he took radiation it might give him a year. It was a big shock for me. Tom was 37 years old at that time, so young so loving. I did not lose my sweet husband. We were unable to decide what to do, as a last hope we went for radiation. About a week of radiation and he felt terrible and lost all of his energy.

We being Christians, went to church for a prayer. Some friends told us of some alternative therapies. People were fighting and winning the battle against cancer. Dr. Johanna Budwig has had and is having success treating cancer patients with her simple protocol. This way we decided to follow this holistic approach which centered on Flax oil and Cottage Cheese in March.

Tom's three month MRI looked good, his brain scan was clean and the hole where they removed the tumor was empty except for a tiny line around a portion of the inside of the hole.

The doctor told that it could be a scar tissue, a benign tumor or a regrowth of the Glioblastoma.

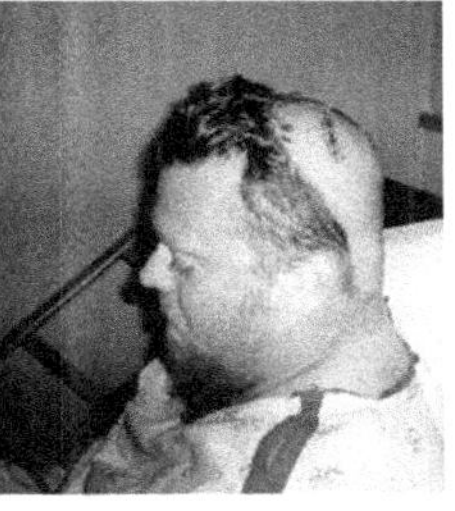

But soon Tom started to recover, began walking for mild exercise and to get some sunlight. We strictly followed the rules and do not eat any pork or fish. It makes it harder for your body to fight cancer if you put unclean and artificial things into it. I think artificial sweetener caused Tom's cancer. He used to drink about 2 liters a day of diet soda every day.

At the six month MRI his brain was completely clean. There was no cancer anywhere. The doctor said that it was a big miracle. In 14 years of practice he had not seen such a healing (CureZone.com).

After 9 months MRI was done in December 2002. He is all right, no sign of any cancer. He started his job and life was back to normal. Praise the Lord Jesus! Dr. Budwig! I am flying in the sky. ☺

Kelly

Healing Story of Jorg Hulf, Hamburg

In September 1980, Jorg Hulf was diagnosed with an adenoid, cystic carcinoma of the tear duct in the left orbital area. He was operated and left eyeball was removed in September 1982. Soon there was a relapse. Again the surgery was performed in the department of oral and maxillofacial surgery in the Oschsenzoll hospital. Doctors told him that his cancer may grow and spread to another eye. So he decided to take the treatment from Dr. Johanna Budwig. Her treatment was scientifically proved, published in medical journals, and is presented at congresses in Germany and abroad (Budwig).

He got the following benefits from using the oil-protein diet and the Eldi oils.

- After surgery the wound healed in a surprisingly short time.
- He had loss of hair in the forehead area, after the first operation. Now hair has grown back in this area.
- He had tooth infection which caused lot of pain, also healed in a short period without ant dental care.
- Blood pressure became normal in a short time and is currently optimal.
- Vision of another eye was improved, from 5.8 previously to the present 4.6.
- He was able to do his job after a short time. He felt very good in body and in mind.
- He frequently suffered from migraine headache before the second operation. His migraine attack was very rare and could be managed without medicines.
- Because his family also strictly taking the oil-protein diet, his wife's chronic constipation vegetative dystonia were cured. Previously, she was treated by doctors for years without success. Similar experiences can also be reported for the children.

How Dr. Budwig saved A. Sch

In early 1993 A. Sch noticed a small growth on the right side of her tongue. Because it was irritating her, she had it surgically removed in the E.N.T. Hospital. Same evening her tongue was swollen and became almost black. She had severe pain and had to be admitted in the hospital for three days. But the doctor assured her that the growth was completely harmless.

After about a week, the hospital told her that she had salivary gland cancer. The growth had already spread in the tongue. A new big operation was suggested under general anesthesia. But she refused to sacrifice her tongue and came back home totally shocked. ☹

She called Dr. Budwig, and took a date for an appointment in the coming week. After meeting Dr. Budwig, she was very much satisfied and cheerful. Meanwhile her family doctor called her to his clinic for a discussion. She went to him. He brutally explained her in harsh words that only removal of 3/4 of the tongue could save her life. She refused for the operation politely. After listening this, he forgot the good manners and he became abusive. He said that she would never survive if she did not go for an operation immediately. She said no, to which he 'shouted: OK then go to hell, no body can help you now. During this entire conversation he did not speak a single word of sympathy. She was completely exhausted and hocked. Every hope of healing was gone. This doctor practically pulled the rug out from under her feet. Totally crushed her husband took her to Dr. Budwig. She wiped her tears and gave her new hope through her special and unique manner and spirit.

The very next day, she started the oil-protein diet explained thoroughly by Dr. Budwig. She used to talk her whenever she needed a support. But threats calls from her family doctor kept coming and soon she became mentally very depressed and sad. She had terrible nightmares. Her husband was hardly able to console her after such nightmares. In the dream she always died under the worst situations she could imagine. Soon she lost interest in everything. This doctor had simply sentenced her to death.

After two years of encouragement and sympathetic touch on the part of Dr. Budwig, the nightmares became less frequent and the fear and anxiety slowly vanished completely. She survived the sickness, thanks to Dr. Budwig. Today she was again a happy and healthy person. The oil-protein diet had done wonderful recovery to her. She was very happy that God sent her to Dr. Budwig. How troublesome a life without a tongue would have been, even if she had survived at all. May God bless Dr. Budwig, the great woman (Budwig).

Ray Schneider

Well I started Budwig FO/CC on September 25, 2016 and the improvement was noted (CT scans) about three months ago so about March. The interval there is six months, but the timing is in part due to the interval between CT scans. I think I'm continuing to improve but I conclude that only because of reduction is pain experience when coughing or sneezing which used to be sharp and excruciating but has now so decline that at most it is only a slight discomfort and seems to be continuing to decline.

Suzanne Johnson

My husband was diagnosed with prostate cancer, so we started the protocol and 3 months later his PSA had dropped to the point that the doctor said you don't have cancer anymore. Still following protocol will have another test in August to see how he is going, but we think it has gone and we are really enjoying the breakfast and lunch mix and eating vegetarian at night. All the best with your cancer

Kathy Maloney Ormsby

My mom (this is her Face book, I don't have one) did Budwig along with her conventional medicine (surgery where they could, chemo and radiation) when she was diagnosed with Adenocarcinoma NSCLC with brain mets. She only did it for a few months and often cheated on the diet part but was consistent with the FOCC. Since then the cancer has been stable until a few weeks ago we learned a tumor might be forming where she had surgery before so she's doing the FOCC mixture about 2-3 times a day and that's almost all she eats because she's not that hungry. The first time around she was on a heavy dose of steroids to help with the swelling in her brain, this made her very hungry. Today the FOCC is enough to be considered a meal. She also eats apricot kernels, randomly and takes at least 200mg of Laetrile a day. Every situation is different but if I had cancer I would stick to the Budwig Protocol 100% along with Apricot kernels. Six years of taking my mom to oncology appointments changed the way I see medicine. I am confused by the way chronic diseases are approached and treated. Well meaning doctors throw Hail Mary's hoping that their prescriptions or surgery will do the trick without any idea or concern about what the patients are eating. And when we asked the DIETITIAN at the oncology clinic she said she had never heard of Budwig or any of the alternative cures we discussed and recommended she stick to the food pyramid and drink Ensure if not hungry.

Lynn Martinez-Mulimbayan

My tumor marker went down about 4 months after I started my Budwig Diet. But I'm doing fruit-vegetable juicing, coffee enema and taking a bunch of supplements as well. At the end of the year, I was able to confirm I was in remission when I had my PET CT scan.

Allie Hayes

I cured my female Siberian Husky 8 and a half years ago of autoimmune disease with the Cottage Cheese Budwig protocol. She was given approx 1 month to live at age 4 , she lived another 6 yrs and only died sadly of unrelated kidney disease (caused by steroids as she got asthma after her autoimmune disease) .Also my sons very close 25 yr old friend took the diet seriously and followed it strictly when he was given six weeks to live with secondary cancers that had spread into his bones . He lived another 7 months on the diet . Doctors were shocked how long he went on for ! It's well worth trying this diet , helps so many things / ailments not just cancers ! Arthritis is another ailment I have seen 95 % proven improvement of in two people !

Ray Schneider

I've been on the Budwig Protocol since about late September last year and had substantial tumor reduction and it didn't hurt. You do have occasional diarrhea as the body gets rid of the waste and you might want to include some detox methods which Johanna Budwig talks about as well. I personally didn't use any detox methods. I read about them in a variety of books, don't remember which particularly. Coffee enemas was one of the most commonly referenced and I think there were a number of others.

Barry Williams

I have been on the Budwig for 12 months, and my Tumor has shrunk 50% and I am feeling fine. I am 75 and still do all the work around the section.

Niti Shah, U.S.A.

Thank you, Dr. Om Verma !! Love your book and the wealth of information you have put it in there so practically! We are going to follow it and live by it thoroughly.... Also deeply appreciate you being so approachable and responsive to the questions we have! It is not always the case. It is almost impossible to find an ethical doctor these days. I think we found one in you! Keep up the good work and sharing your knowledge with all of us.... I also connected with one of your patient who had a complete recovery from a stage 4 cancer and amazed to hear the patient side of the healing journey! Blessings and best of health.

My Cancer journey with Dr O P Verma and his great book

Hello, my name is Dawne and I live in United States. I am here to share you my cancer experience with Dr Verma's book "Cancer Cause And Cure". It really helped me along my journey. The first three months after I got my diagnosis I was all over the place, I was reading books, I was listening to videos, and I was searching TV, anything and everything that has to do with cancer. One of the biggest problem that I faced was that I was very lonely, I was very afraid and my Oncologist didn't make things better. She was extremely negative and her only way of saying that she was going to cure me was chemo, radiation and surgery. I am on the other hand did not believe in chemo, radiation and surgery. It may have a place in some people but not in my life. I knew that I have to do this through a more holistic natural way. Every part of my body kept telling me not to do chemo and radiation, that there was another way for me and of course I expressed this to my Oncologist and that was a mistake, because she was very negative, she attacked me verbally, calling me a fool, that I am going to die the worst death ever and it was terrifying, it was very scaring.

Like I said, in the First three months I was doing intense research, research of my life and I did a lot of things to heal my cancer and I took everything whatever told me to do it, I did it. I was that afraid so the good news is I must be doing something right when pray to my creator and I ask please guide me in the way, you know you made me, you know how to fix me and undo all the damage that I did to my body because I know I am the one who caused this cancer.

Yes, I have support of my family. Nobody in my family had cancer that knew what to do. So the support they gave me was whatever I decided they would back me up they wouldn't fight me because it is my life. And even I get love from my family I was so alone I was so afraid. Then finally after I was diagnosed I came across a very important book. Oh my goodness, I wish somebody has given me this book at first. It is besides my Bible my creator's word, I consider this my second Bible. The Second most important book in my life and we all know that doctor who wrote this. This is very important to me, but called "Cancer Cause And Cure" and this book really pulled it all together for me. That's the one book that hit me here right in my heart. If I find anybody in my life or if anybody talks about cancer that's the book I am taking him to. It saved my life. It saved my sanity. It kept me from going crazy, wandering, terrified. It was the book that gave me lot of hope. Like I said I don't believe in chemo and radiation. I was already toxic that's why I had cancer, so why I want to put more toxins in my body. The book gave me a lot of reassurance and guidance and that's what I needed. No other book that I had read and believe me I read a lot of books, no other book was as informative as the Cancer Cause And Cure. One of the things about the book in the beginning that it talks about the topic of cancer and two doctor's works, they explain very simply why we get cancer, why I had got cancer and that's the one thing a lot of western medical doctors here in United States won't talk about it. Don't worry how you got? You got it let's cut it out, lets burn it out. And I was before that and I didn't understand scientific medical journals I am not a doctor. I tried to read those book, they terrified me they put me to sleep and I didn't understand what they were talking about. At least with Dr Verma's book I was able to understand a lot of words written there and at least I can work with that. He speaks about the Budwig, the German doctor and that's why I started in the beginning because my sister and I had talked about it a year ago. It's funny, we talked what would we do if we get cancer and we had talked about the Budwig Protocol and once I got my message from my doctor that I had cancer that's the first thing that came into my head Budwig and I read one of Budwig's book. And it helped me learn about what I am supposed to do, but Dr Verma's book made it just a little bit easier to understand because he explains a lot. I was doing the Budwig but I was not doing it quite right, my timing was off. So his book showed me how I am supposed to do it and I got the timing right and another thing with Dr Verma, I thank you so much for being on Face book because whenever I had questions, I was able to ask him you know specific question there and he was so gracious to answer my questions. You know a lot of things when you start doing the Budwig and don't have correct information, you don't really understand how you are supposed to do it correct. Lot of people don't do sauerkraut juice, lot of people don't do teas and champagne. I started to understand this and I made it part of my protocol. I was doing it at first, but I was not doing it completely right. And lot of other things western medical doctors here tell you that there a sun, sun is bad for you causes cancer. Budwig didn't say that. She said you needed it. You need sun, it is important. And Dr Verma's book reiterated that and lot of other therapies that I didn't know about. Some therapies that I was doing were the enemas and again I was not doing it quite right until I got Dr Verma's book. And it explains me that how and what I had to do and I also learned about soaks thorough his book, bath soaks and how to do it? How long to do it? What you should be putting in your bath tubs? Why it is important to do these bath soaks? Another thing that I learned was about supplements. How important they were? And foods you stay away from meats. I used to be a big meat eater. Not anymore no thank you no no no. I have thrown away meat and I eat raw vegetables, fruits, nuts and seeds. That is the base of my diet and I learned that a lot about the Budwig Protocol and other therapies that the book covers. And about pain therapies, I did not know that you can help with pain certain supplements or certain just regular foods. And by Turmeric, Turmeric did a lot for me, it helped in my detox.

And another thing is not in just cancer but diabetes, I used to be, I am type 2 diabetic. I was always told that I will never stop type 2 diabetes. I used to take insulin I used to take pills. With the diet I am on and the ways that I followed the Cancer Cause And Cure book, I no longer have to take medicines for diabetes and also no longer high cholesterol. So the book is wonderful as far as helping me in cancer but helping me in other issues. I also learned to do the mental exercises that the book covers and physical exercises . I am very limited in my abilities to do certain exercises. I walk with the cane. I have my back many years ago. But the exercises they talk in the book taught me how to do things to help my cancer, how to get lymph nodes cleared, how to get lymph system moving and also meditation, I never meditated in my life. And I realize the importance of meditation because he wrote in his book. Also organ cleanses liver cleanses, kidney cleanse and even parasite cleanse. I never thought to do parasite cleanse until I got hold of Dr. Verma's book.

I am glad that he also introduced Lothar Hirneise I read in the book how he was successful in healing patients and that he actually knew Dr Budwig that was so important for me. One of the thing that Lothar covers is the Tumor, how here in United State they will cut the tumor out. And of the thing he specifically says don't do that. Tumor is very important and all along before I even read that I was taught the tumor is just not the cancer, not just the cancer itself, there was more to it, I thought like the tumor was there for important reason, I just don't understand why? But Dr Lothar did and that was good enough for me. And there were many other therapies that other doctors talk about in the book specially dealing with emotions. How emotions help with your past experience and also dealing with people in your life, people that are positive and good for you, but also getting rid of negative people. The first person I got negative was my oncologist. After 3 visits, even when my tumor was shrinking she kept saying you are going die, you are going to die, you have to do this, you have to do chemo, and you have to do radiation. I finally said enough is enough. And I just got off with her. I had another oncologist who is open minded enough. When I told him about what I was doing with the Cancer Cause And Cure and I found Internal Medicine doctor who is integrative, he believes in holistic healing.

One of the thing about The Cancer Cause And Cure book is that you gain an immediate understanding what you got to do. And after first three months I was but once I got the book I followed exactly what it said . I noticed a big difference. First of all I was so calm, I was so relaxed and I put a lot of faith into the book. I now I put my faith in the right ways. This book, you know teaches you how to make the time your friend and the first three months time was not my friend. I thought time was against me. With the book I got to use my time wisely. I don't waste any more time on research. Once I got the Cancer Cause And Cure book that was the end of my research. I knew that I did the right thing by getting the book. And like I said I don't believe Cancer Cause And Cure book is not just for the people with cancer, it's for many other reasons, I feel so much healthier, so much happier.

So Dr Verma from the bottom of my heart, to the top of my heart and throw out my heart, I thank you, I thank you so much for saving my sanity saving my life because the tests that are coming back keep saying that everything is good Sine May and November and I had two tests in between my blood is still clean there is no tumor and there are no swollen nodes and I thank you thank you for being there thank you for writing the book so with that I say farewell you take care and people listen to the book it will save your life Thank you and bless you. Take care…

Mrs Dawne Ulvano U S A

Lucie Bois cured her Breast Cancer by Budwig

I shrunk à big tumor (8.5 cm) in my right breast using Essiac and Budwig protocol. plus lots of fresh homemade veggies juices, organic products, coffee enemas and much more. You got to be committed to à very healthy lifestyle to heal safely.

The tumor has shrunk and could barely be detected on my last Doppler ultrasound test last September and my tumor markers went back into normal range. It took me 2 years and à half to be there. My only challenge now is cancer metastasized as Paget disease of the nipple. Long journey some would say. It would be too long to explain all the protocols I've used (and still using) just on a text. I could say that I used à quite Big arsenal against cancer. Everything God has provide in His nature and non-toxic scientific methods.   I never took chemotherapy, radiations nor any surgery.

159

Prayer and my faith in à good God who wants the best for me. When you know that you are loved deeply by Creator of the universe who came on earth in the person of Jesus, it gives me assurance. I am also persuaded that God is very unpleased with the corruption in the actual medical system and is raising à squad of uncorrupt Ph.D. and survivors who Will show à different way to heal while respecting the Law of Nature. Now I have a very good reason to heal. It is à mission.

Lucie Bois
Dec 15, 2016

Alisha D'Mello cured her mom's uterine cancer

Hello Dr Verma, thank you for your inspiration and guidance. My mother who has uterine cancer has started the budwig protocol. She is using 2% organic Cottage Cheese as this is what is available to us. Thank you in advance. Alisha

Posted on Jan 26, 2016

Hello everyone. Wanted to give an update on mom and share some positivity. She was diagnosed with uterine cancer one year ago..with liver met. Chemo was offered but she declined. Started juicing, doing the budwig protocol, cut out meat dairy and sugar, coffee enemas, light exercise and prayer. Liver met was stable after 3 months, started shrinking after another 3 months. She got results for her CT scan today (its been 6 months since the last one) and all clear! She will continue with her diet indefinitely.

Alisha D'Mello
Posted on Dec 17, 2016
(https://www.facebook.com/groups/budwig)

The Budwig Diet quotes

"What she (Dr. Johanna Budwig) has demonstrated to my initial disbelief but lately, to my complete satisfaction in my practice is: CANCER IS EASILY CURABLE, the treatment is dietary/lifestyle, the response is immediate; the cancer cell is weak and vulnerable; the precise biochemical breakdown point was identified by her in 1951 and is specifically correctable, in vitro (test-tube) as well as in vivo (real)... "

Dr. Dan C. Roehm M.D. FACP (Oncologist and former cardiologist) in 1990

"Cancer patients suffer from a faulty metabolism caused by a malfunction in the lipid defense system. By repairing the lipid defense system the cancer cannot survive. Of course common chemo and radiation causes further harm to the lipid defense system -- the very system that protects you from cancer! The folks who will READILY ADMIT that they don't understand the cancer mechanism will tell you with their next breath that cancer can be killed with poisons. So can you. Would you trust your car to a so-called mechanic who didn't understand what makes a car work properly? If not, why would you let someone who doesn't understand cancer "fix" your body? The average cancer docs don't know - they admit it. That doesn't make them bad people; it just makes them unqualified to treat your condition if you have cancer. Don't let unqualified people poison you just because they don't know what else to do".

William Kelley Eidem, author "The Doctor Who Cures Cancer (Dr Revici)

"To sell chemotherapy as 'therapy' is most likely the biggest deceit in the history of medicine. Whoever masterminded this chemo-torture deserves a monument in the hell."

Dr. Ryke Geerd Hamer

"I have the answer to cancer, but American doctors won't listen. They come here and observe my methods and are impressed. Then they want to make a special deal so they can take it home and make a lot of money. I won't do it, so I'm blackballed in every country."

Dr Budwig

Dr Rudin believes the Omega 3 story parallels the story of Beriberi & Pellagra. It took them 200 years to accept pellagra was a nutrient deficiency.

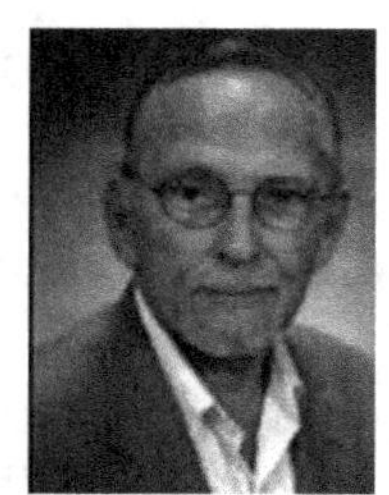

"Nobody seemed to notice that a crime has been committed: It was the case of the missing nutrient. The nutrient was essential; it was a nutrient we human beings needed in order to stay healthy. It started to disappear from our diet about 75 years ago and now is almost gone. Only about 20% of the amount needed for human health and well-being remains. The nutrient is a fatty acid so important and so little understood that I call it "the nutritional missing link"….Food grade linseed oil & fish oil are the best sources of this special fat—Omega 3 essential fatty acid—which modern food destroys."

Donaldo Rudin, M.D. (The Omega 3 Phenomenon)

In a 1994 study of 121 women with breast cancer, those in more advanced stages whose breast cancer had spread to their lymph nodes showed the lowest levels of omega-3 fatty acids in the breast tissue. After 31 months, the 20 women who had developed metastases had significantly lower levels of these EFAs (Essential fatty acids) than those who didn't. Another study out of Boston University using the same type of tissue profiles that were used in the breast cancer study demonstrated that patients with coronary artery disease likewise had low levels of EFAs.

"The association between fats—meaning saturated, refined w6s (Omega 6), rancid fats, processed oils, and altered fats---and cancer, (but excluding w3s and fresh, natural, unrefined oils) has long been documented. (They) interfere with oxygen use in our cells. Heat, hydrogenation, light, and oxygen produce chemically altered fat products that are toxic to our cells....These fats kill people. Healing fats in cancer include...... Omega 3s, enhance oxygen use in cells, decrease tumor formation, slow tumor growth, decrease tumor formation, decrease the spread of cancer cells (metastasis), and extend the patient's survival time. Unsaturated fatty acids in fresh, unheated oils are anti-mutagenic. Saturated fatty acids to not have this protective ability. Heating these oils above 150^0 C makes them lose their protective power, and they become mutation-causing. ALL mass market oils except virgin olive oil have undergone heating during deodorization...When we use virgin olive oil or other unrefined oils for sautéing; frying...we overheat them, destroying their protective, anti-mutagenic properties. ALL hydrogenated and partially hydrogenated products have also been overheated.."

Udo Erasmus (Fats That Heal, Fats That Kill)

"Our immune system, which is vital for destroying cancer cells, requires EFAs, vitamins C, B6, and A, and zinc to function, and requires an exceptionally rich nutrient supply of ALL essential nutrients for its high level of complex cellular activities. Deficiencies of EFAs and toxic, man-made synthetic drugs that interfere with essential fatty acid functions can create the conditions of fatty degeneration collectively known as cancer."

Udo Erasmus

"Compared to 100 years ago, Omega 3 is down 80%, B vitamins are estimated to be down to about 50% of the daily requirement. Vitamin B6 consumption may be low as it is removed in grain milling and not replaced. Vitamins B1, B2, B3 and E have also been lost in food processing. Minerals are depleted in a similar way. Fiber is down 75-80%. Ant nutrients have increased substantially---saturated fat, 100%; cholesterol,

50%; refined sugar nearly 1000%; salt up to 500%; and funny fat isomers nearly 1,000%."

Dr Rudin

Dr. Johanna Budwig is rightly known far beyond the borders of Germany. Her ingenious, simple, and effective oil-protein diet has found adherents throughout the world and it has helped many people to particularly better deal with their cancer illness.

I had the great good fortune of spending many days in discussion with her over a period of several years, of being able to study her extensive case histories, of giving joint presentations with her, and of thus gaining an understanding of nutrition for myself that extended far beyond that which I was previously able to find in the usual literature. But what was most convincing to me in my activity on the executive board of Menschen gegen Krebs in Germany was the oil-protein diet.

Hardly a day goes by when I do not talk with people on the phone that has changed their diet along the guidelines provided by Dr. Budwig. I am party first-hand to how successful this nutrition therapy is. I consciously use the term nutrition therapy and not cancer diet because I think it would be an injustice to Dr. Budwig to not to distinguish her scientifically grounded oil-protein therapy from all the diets that are offered around the world.

For me the oil-protein diet always serves as the basis of a cancer therapy and please understands that I am not just simply writing this, but that I have carefully chosen my words, as I have become familiar with more than 100 different alternative cancer therapies in recent years, and I have investigated many of them. When Dr. Johanna Budwig died the cancer scene lost one of the last great scientists of the last century, and it behooves each of us to carry her legacy to future generations, so that they as well can profit from the oil-protein diet.

Lothar Hirneise

I am referring to a super nutrient, which has been neglected for decades, it is neither taught properly in the schools, nor the doctors discuss about it openly, multinationals have removed this from our diet, but the hard truth is that it is essential for our body, it keeps us healthy and fit, protects us from many serious ailments, its presence is essential for cellular respiration, our cells suffocate in its absence, without this our life is impossible, name of this nutrient is alpha-linolenic acid, which is head of the omega-3 family and the richest food source is FLAX SEED OIL.

Dr. O.P. Verma, Flax Guru

They (American Cancer Society) lie like scoundrels.

M. Dean Burk PhD who worked for the National Cancer Institute for 34 years

There have been many cancer cures, and all have been ruthlessly and systematically suppressed with a Gestapo-like thoroughness by the cancer establishment.

Robert C. Atkins MD

Essiac Is A Cure For Cancer. I've seen it reverse and eliminate cancers at such a progressed state that nothing medical science currently has could have accomplished similar results. I wouldn't have believed it myself had I not seen it with my own eyes. I feel very strongly that Essiac is the single most beneficial treatment for cancer today.

C.A. Brusch, M.D., J.F.K's personal physician talking to radio talk show host and producer Elaine Alexander in a radio broadcast from Vancouver, British Columbia, in November 1984

The War Against Quackery is a carefully orchestrated, heavily endowed campaign sponsored by extremists holding positions of power in the orthodox hierarchy.....The multimillion-dollar campaign against quackery was never meant to root out incompetent doctors; it was, and is, designed specifically to destroy alternative medicine...The millions were raised and spent because orthodox medicine sees alternative, drugless medicine as a real threat to its economic power. And right they are...the majority of the drug houses will not survive.

Dr Atkins, M.D. (The Healing of Cancer by Barry Lynes)

And what do I actually do? I give cancer patients simple, natural foods. That is all. I take sick people out of the hospital, when it is said there that they do not have more than an hour or two left to live, that the scientifically attested diagnosis is at hand and that the patient is completely moribund. In most cases I can help even these patients quickly and conclusively.

Dr. Johanna Budwig, in "Flax Oil as a True Aid"

Cancer has only one prime cause. It is the replacement of normal oxygen respiration of the body's cells by an anaerobic (i.e., oxygen-deficient) cell respiration.

Dr. Otto Warburg, twice Nobel Laureate

...the cause of cancer is no longer a mystery; we know it occurs whenever any cell is denied 60% of its oxygen requirements.

Cancer, above all other diseases, has countless secondary causes. But, even for cancer, there is only one prime cause. Summarized in a few words, the prime cause of cancer is the replacement of the respiration of oxygen in normal body cells by a fermentation of sugar. All normal body cells meet their energy needs by respiration of oxygen, whereas cancer cells meet their energy needs in great part by fermentation. All normal body cells are thus obligate aerobes, whereas all cancer cells are partial anaerobes.

Dr. Otto Warburg Prime Cause and Prevention of Cancer

[C]hemotherapy is basically ineffective in the vast majority of cases in which it is given.

Ralph Moss, PhD, former Director of Information for Sloan Kettering Cancer Research Center

Three Australian oncologists - Associate Professor Graeme Morgan, Professor Robyn Ward and Dr. Michael Barton - undertook a meta-analysis aiming to determine the actual contribution of cytotoxic chemotherapy to survival in adult cancer patients. Their results, published in "Clinical Oncology" in 2004 under the title "The contribution of cytotoxic chemotherapy to 5-year survival in adult malignancies" (abstract available at www.ncbi.nlm.nih.gov/pubmed/15630849) found the overall contribution of these drugs to 5-year survival in adults to be an estimated 2.3% in Australia and 2.1% in the USA. See Table: Impact of cytotoxic chemotherapy on 5-year survival in American adults showing the percentage of 5-year survivors after chemotherapy for 22 types of cancer. The authors concluded that "it is clear that cytotoxic chemotherapy only makes a minor contribution to cancer survival".

A detailed review of this important paper is owed to Dr. Ralph Moss and can be read for instance at www.icnr.com/articles/ischemotherapyeffective.html under the title "How Effective Is Chemo Therapy?"

Healing Cancer Naturally

"Best book I've ever read on chemotherapy."

Ralph Moss' Questioning Chemotherapy is a book that every person faced with cancer must read before submitting to toxic chemicals which may very well destroy the body's immune system. Unlike many alternative health authors who base their conclusions on anecdotal evidence, Moss uses the medical establishment's own research to prove that in almost all instances chemotherapy is NOT a viable approach to improving cancer survival rates. Moss also makes the important point that current cancer research has never bothered to examine the mental anguish, physical suffering, and poor quality of life endured by almost everyone whose doctors talk or scare them into undergoing chemotherapy. Learning about the economics behind chemotherapy drives the final nail into the coffin of a "therapy" that educated people in the future will consider outrageous and reflective of the current dark ages of so-called modern medicine. This is a must read book for anyone who wants to know the truth behind chemotherapy or anyone whose doctor wants to inject toxic chemicals into their bloodstream.

Chet Day's review of "Questioning Chemotherapy: A Critique of the Use of Toxic Drugs in the Treatment of Cancer" by Ralph W. Moss

Except for two forms of cancer, chemotherapy does not cure. It tortures and may shorten life...

Dr. Candace Pert, Georgetown University

Chemo drugs are some of the most toxic substances ever designed to go into a human body, their effects are very serious, and are often the direct cause of death. Like the case of Jackie Onassis, who underwent chemo for one of the rare diseases in which it generally has some beneficial results: non-Hodgkin's lymphoma. She went into the hospital on Friday and was dead by Tuesday.

Dr Tim O'Shea in TO THE CANCER PATIENT

Cancer researchers, medical journals, and the popular media all have contributed to a situation in which many people with common malignancies are being treated with drugs not known to be effective.

Dr. Martin Shapiro UCLA

Disclaimer

This book is not intended to replace the advice and/or care of a qualified health care professional. Please do not try to self diagnose or self treat any disease. Seek professional help and consult your physician before making any dietary changes.

This book is not intended to provide medical advice and is sold with the understanding that the publisher and the author have neither liability nor responsibility to any person or entity with respect to loss, damage or injury caused or alleged to be caused directly or indirectly by the information contained in this book or the use of any products mentioned. Readers should not use any of the product discussed in this book without the advice of a medical profession.

The Food and Drug Administration has not approved the use of any of the natural treatments discussed in this book. This book, and the information contained herein, has not been approved by the Food and the Drug Administration.

Bibliography

MNT Knowledge Center.com. (n.d.). Retrieved from http://www.medicalnewstoday.com/articles/265990.php

Nobelprize.org. (n.d.). Retrieved from http://www.nobelprize.org/nobel_prizes/medicine/laureates/1931/warburg-bio.html

About Health. (n.d.). Retrieved from http://lowcarbdiets.about.com/od/nutrition/a/fiberbenefits.htm

Acids, O. F. (n.d.). Retrieved from http://themedicalbiochemistrypage.org/omegafats.php

American Nutrition Association. (1972). Retrieved from http://americannutritionassociation.org/newsletter/Flax seed-neglected-food

Ben Green Field Fitness. (n.d.). Retrieved from http://www.bengreenfieldfitness.com/2014/06/bulletproof-coffee-enema/

Budwig, D. J. Cancer The Problem And The Solution.

Budwig, D. J. FlaxOil As A True Aid Against Arthritis, Heart Infarction, Cancer, And Other Diseases .

Budwig, D. J. (1994). *The Oil-Protein Diet Cookbook*. Vancouver, Canada: Apple Publishing Co. Ltd.

Cairns, G. (n.d.). *Cancer Tutor.com*. Retrieved from http://www.cancertutor.com/dandelionroot/

Canada, F. C. (n.d.). Retrieved from http://www.Flaxcouncil.ca/english/pdf/FlxPrmr_4ed_Chpt2.pdf

Craig, G. (March 15, 2011). *The EFT Manual Paperback*.

CureZone.com. (n.d.). *CureZone.com*. Retrieved from http://curezone.com/forums/am.asp?i=67355

Doctor NDTV. (n.d.). Retrieved from http://doctor.ndtv.com/faq/ndtv/fid/20230/Are_Flax_seeds_benef icial_for_osteoarthritis_patients.html

Dr Robert E. Willner M.D., P. (1993). *THE CANCER SOLUTION* .

Dr. Johanna Budwig Stiftung . (n.d.). Retrieved from http://www.budwig-stiftung.de/dr-johanna-budwig/ihr-leben.html

Escher, U. (n.d.). *BudwigDVDs.com*. Retrieved from http://www.budwigdvds.com/articles/budwig-diet-protocol-videos.htm

Euler, L. (n.d.). *Cancer Defeated.com*. Retrieved from http://www.cancerdefeated.com/newsletters/Plant-that-Cures-Practically-Everything.html

Feast without fear.com. (n.d.). Retrieved from https://feastwithoutfear.wordpress.com/2012/12/01/understanding -omega-3-and-omega-6-pathways-how-it-could-change-your-life/

Hamer, D. R. CANCER, DISEASE OF THE PSYCHE.

Healing Cancer Naturally . (n.d.). Retrieved from http://www.healingcancernaturally.com/lymphedema-treatment-therapy.html

Healing Cancer Naturally . (n.d.). Retrieved from http://www.healingcancernaturally.com/chemotherapy-nausea-vomiting.html

healingcancernaturally.com. (n.d.). Retrieved from http://www.healingcancernaturally.com/budwig-treatment-advice-very-ill-patients.html

Healingcancernaturally.com. (n.d.). Retrieved from http://www.healingcancernaturally.com/cancer-pain-management-relief.html

Health Freedom.com. (n.d.). Retrieved from http://www.healthfreedom.info/sheep_sorrel.htm

Hirneise, L. (2005). *Chemotherapy Heals Cancer And World Is Flat* (Vol. 1). Germany: www.nexus-health.com.

https://en.wikipedia.org/wiki/Otto_Heinrich_Warburg. (n.d.). Retrieved from Wikipedia.

ICRF Independent Cancer Research Foundation, I. L. (n.d.). *Cancer Tutor.com*. Retrieved from http://www.cancertutor.com/black_cumin/

Minarsich, M. (n.d.). *Bionatures* . Retrieved from http://bionaturesblog.com/

Minarsich, M. (n.d.). *http://budwigFlax.blogspot.in/*. Retrieved from BioNatures Blog: http://budwigFlax.blogspot.in/

ND, F. B. (n.d.). *Healthy.net*. Retrieved from http://www.healthy.net/Health/Article/Treatment_of_Coughs_Wi th_Herbal_Remedies/774/2.

ND, F. B. (n.d.). *Healthy.net*. Retrieved from http://www.healthy.net/Health/Article/Treatment_of_Coughs_Wi th_Herbal_Remedies/774/3

Olson, S. (n.d.). *Budwig Videos.com*. Retrieved from http://www.budwig-videos.com/categories/20071009_3

Osburn, L. (n.d.). *Seeds of Longevity and a New Golden Age*. Retrieved from http://alchemylab.com/seeds_of_a_new_gold.htm

Paradise, V. i. (n.d.). Retrieved from http://www.vegparadise.com/highestperch53.html

Philip E.Bizel, M. (n.d.). *Alive and Well* .

PR Web. (n.d.). Retrieved from http://www.prweb.com/releases/AIDS/2007/prweb572849.htm

Puna Wai Ora Mind-Body Cancer Clinic . (2006-2014). Retrieved from http://www.alternative-cancer-care.com/dr-ryke-geerd-hamer.html

S.A.Wilsons.com. (n.d.). Retrieved from http://www.sawilsons.com/coffee.htm

Schmid, U. (n.d.). *Healing Cancer Naturally*. Retrieved from http://www.healingcancernaturally.com/budwigcompatiblepainm anagement.html

Schmid, U. (n.d.). *Healing Cancer Naturally*. Retrieved from http://www.healingcancernaturally.com/warburgcancer-cause-prevention.html

Skelton, C. (n.d.). *The Budwig Diet / Protocol*. Retrieved from http://www.budwig-diet.co.uk/eldi-oils/

Wikipedia. (n.d.). Retrieved from https://en.wikipedia.org/wiki/Otto_Heinrich_Warburg

Index

Awesome Flax: A Book by Flax Guru [Kindle Edition]

http://www.amazon.com/Awesome-Flax-Book-Guru-ebook/dp/B00PUUIR0K

Book Description

Flax seed- Miraculous Anti-ageing Divine Food

What is Flax seed and how can it benefit me? I was faced with this question when I started hearing about Flax seed not long ago. It became a 'buzz word' in society and seems to be making great role in increased health for many. I wanted to join that wagon of wellness and so I researched until I felt satisfied that it could help me, too. Here are my findings.

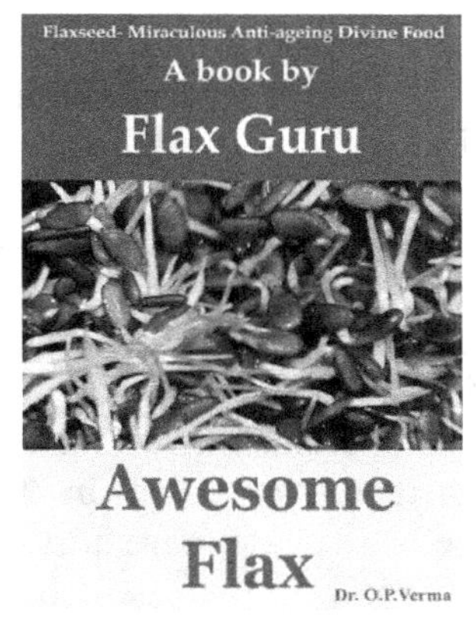

Flax seeds are the hard, tiny seeds of Linum usitatissimum, the Flax plant, which has been widely used for thousands of years as a source of food and clothing. Flax seeds have become very popular recently, because they are a richest source of the Omega 3 essential fatty acid; also known as Alpha Linolenic Acid (ALA) and lignans. People in the new millennium may see Flax seed as an important new FOOD SUPER STAR. In fact, there's nobody who won't benefit by adding Flax seed to his or her diet. Even Gandhi wrote: "Wherever Flax seed becomes a regular food item among the people, there will be better health."

Flax seed contains 30-40% oil (including 36-50% alpha linolenic acid, 23-24% linoleic acid- Omega-6 fatty acids and oleic acids), mucilage (6%), protein (25%), Vitamin B group, lecithin, selenium, calcium, folate, magnesium, zinc, iron, carotene, sulfur, potassium, phosphorous, manganese, silicon, copper, nickel, molybdenum, chromium, and cobalt, vitamins A and E and all essential amino acids.

Other fatty acids, omega-6's, is abundant in vegetable oils such as corn, soybean, safflower, and sunflower oils as well as in the many processed foods made from these oils. Omega-6 fatty acids have stimulating, irritating and inflammatory effect while omega-3 fatty acids have calming and soothing effect on our body. Our bodies function best when our diets contain a well-balanced ratio of these fatty acids, meaning 1:1 to 4:1 of omega-6 and omega-3. But we typically eat 10 to 30 times more omega-6's than omega-3's, which is a prescription for trouble. This imbalance puts us at greater risk for a number of serious illnesses, including heart disease, cancer, stroke, and arthritis. As the most abundant plant source of omega-3 fatty acids, Flax seed helps restore balance and lets omega-3's do what they're best at: balancing the immune system, decreasing inflammation, and lowering some of the risk factors for heart disease.

One way that Omega 3 essential fatty acid known as Alpha Linolenic Acid ALA helps the heart is by decreasing the ability of platelets to clump together. Flax seed helps to lower high blood pressure, clears clogged coronaries, lowers high blood cholesterol, bad LDL cholesterol and triglyceride levels and raises good HDL cholesterol. It can relieve the symptoms of Diabetes Mellitus. It lowers blood sugar level. Flax seed help fight obesity. Adding Flax seed to foods creates a feeling of satiation. Furthermore, Flax seed stokes the metabolic processes in our cells. Much like a furnace, once stoked, the cells generate more heat and burn calories.

Flax seeds are the most abundant source of lignans. Lignans are plant-based compounds that can block estrogen activity in cells, reducing the risk of Breast, Uterus, Colon and Prostate cancers. According to the US Department of Agriculture, Flax seed contains 27 identifiable cancer preventative compounds. Lignans in Flax seeds are 200 to 800 times more than any other lignan source. Lignans are phytoestrogens, meaning that they are similar to but weaker than the estrogen that a woman's body produces naturally. Therefore, they may also help alleviate menopausal discomforts such as hot flashes and vaginal dryness. They are also antibacterial, antifungal, and antiviral.

Because they are high in dietary fiber, ground Flax seeds can help ease the passage of stools and thus relieve constipation, hemorrhoids and diverticular disease. Taken for inflammatory bowel disease, Flax seed can help to calm inflammation and repair any intestinal tract damage.